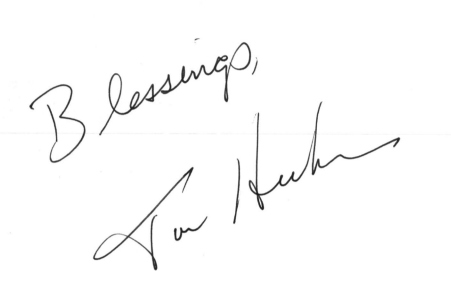

Leaving the fear of
breast cancer behind

Journey to Hope

A book of self-care
and prevention for women
and the men who love them

Thomas Hudson, MD

Cathee A. Poulsen, Editor

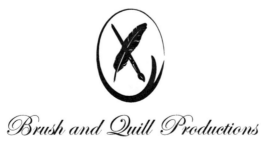

Brush and Quill Productions
Naples, Florida
USA

Every effort has been made to make this book as accurate as possible. Any errors or inconsistencies are unintentional. The purpose of this book is to inform and educate. No individual should use the information in this book for self-diagnosis, treatment or as justification for accepting or declining any medical therapy for any health problem or disease. No individual is discouraged from seeking professional medical advice and treatment. This book is not supplying medical advice. Any application of the information herein is at the reader's own risk. Any individual with a specific health problem or who is taking medication should first seek advice from his or her personal physician or healthcare provider before starting any program of self-care, especially one that includes a change in diet or level of exercise.

Published by:
Brush and Quill Productions First Paperback Edition 2011
www.BrushandQuillProductions.com
Naples, Florida

Printed by Lightning Source , Inc., an Ingram Content Company
1246 Heil Quaker Blvd.
La Vergne, TN USA 37086

ISBN 978-0-615-44276-1
Library of Congress Control Number: 2011921732

Editing by Cathee A. Poulsen
Cover and book layout by Sue Riger
Cover photo collage by Sue Riger includes:
    bridge photo by FireBrandPhotography © istockphoto.com;
    and woman photo by RedBarnStudio © istockphoto.com

To order this book from the author, please visit
www.YourJourneytoHope.com/book.html

To Sharron

We Miss You

&

About the Author

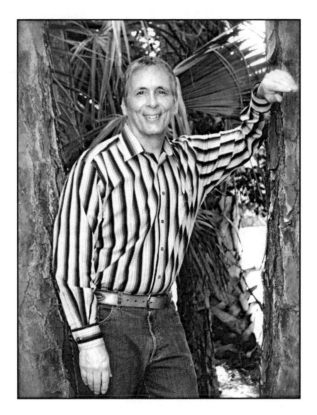

Dr. Thomas Hudson is a diagnostic radiologist specializing in mammography and breast imaging. He attended medical school at the University of Maryland in Baltimore, and completed his radiology residency at Walter Reed Army Medical Center in Washington, D.C. After his time in the Army he settled in Naples FL, where he served as Director of Women's Imaging at Naples Diagnostic Imaging Centers (NDIC). Since 2005, Dr. Hudson has been an independent women's imaging consultant, most recently at the prestigious Women's Center for Radiology in Orlando, FL. He is also on the faculty of the Center for Mind-Body Medicine in Washington, D.C. His passion is to educate women about self-care as it relates to breast cancer and breast cancer prevention. He lectures to larger groups as well as counsels women one on one about a mind-body-spirit approach to their health.

Table of Contents

Table of Contents

Foreword

James S. Gordon, MD, a psychiatrist, is the founder and director of The Center for Mind-Body Medicine, and the author of *Comprehensive Cancer Care: Integrating Complementary, Conventional and Alternative Therapies* and, most recently, of *Unstuck: Your Guide to the Seven Stage Journey Out of Depression.*

I met Tom Hudson seven or eight years ago at our CancerGuides training, the Center for Mind-Body Medicine program that teaches cancer specialists, other health professionals, and patient advocates how to help people with cancer create comprehensive and integrative programs of care. We present talks on how mind-body approaches like meditation, guided imagery, nutrition and exercise, Chinese medicine, and group support can all help people with cancer to live longer and better. We also conduct small groups where our students explore their attitudes toward cancer and its treatment, as well as death and dying. In group, they share their feelings about their work, their experiences, and their hopes and fears, with one another.

Tom Hudson was in my small group along with ten others—a couple of oncologists, as cancer specialists are called, some other doctors and researchers, several oncology nurses, an acupuncturist and some psychotherapists who work primarily with cancer patients and their families.

Everyone was smart and curious, determined to learn as much as they could and bring back new kinds of help to their patients. There was, however, something about Tom's intelligence and curiosity that set him apart. An openness to learning new science and new ways of looking at standard treatments that was total and uncompromising. A willingness to revise what he had long believed. Tom had the courage to consider changing fundamental ways he had practiced, as long as it made sense and could make a difference to his patients.

Along with his intelligence, curiosity, and commitment to his patients' welfare, there was something else I, and everyone in the group, quickly recognized—Tom's kindness. It's a quality most of us didn't associate with diagnostic radiologists, who can often seem like remote, dispassionate observers, not engaged and friendly clinicians. We could feel Tom's kindness in the way he listened to us share our struggles, and hear it in the words he spoke—not facile attempts to show us he understood, but a deep sharing of how what we said and who we were had touched him. How our concerns brought up struggles and challenges he had faced. How our words had helped him understand himself better, even as they brought him closer to us. I'm quite sure everyone in that group felt known and appreciated by Tom.

I'm just as sure that as you read *Journey to Hope* you will feel the same kindness. As a scientist who has devoted much of his career to the subtleties of mammography, Tom has taken a long and highly informed look at what we know, and what we don't know about breast cancer, its treatment and prevention. He explains to you with great care, clarity, and sensitivity, what you need to know. You'll feel that he is there with you and your loved ones as you navigate the confusing, perilous journey through cancer and its treatment.

You will find new information here that will help you live better, and perhaps longer, with breast cancer. Some of this information you may have heard before, but is presented here in a voice—gentle, friendly, and personal—that will allow you to hear it in a new way. You may find in this book the knowledge and confidence to make the wisest choices in your own care, and the courage, even in the face of the dogma that sometimes passes for wisdom, to chart a course that will help you to heal.

Much of what you will learn in *Journey to Hope* may surprise you. Tom points out, for instance, that contrary to what most people believe, and what many physicians convey to their patients, breast cancer is more than just a genetic disease. There are many factors involved in breast cancer risk, a number of which—diet, exercise, stress, attitude, and social support—you can do something about. There are perspectives and practices, as Tom explains, that can help prevent breast cancer and also help to more successfully, along with conventional therapies, treat it. He shows us, step by simple, clear step, exactly what we can do to put our bets on the side of good health and longer life.

The practical information in *Journey to Hope* is enormously valuable, but the title of the book hints at even greater, less obvious, riches. It is a reservoir of understanding that can help women find strength and healing in the face of the most daunting challenges. Like the good writer he is, Tom doesn't just tell us how, he shows us, through stories about people he has known and cared for, and by sharing the painful, deeply instructive, learning of his own life.

Over the last eight years I've come to know Tom Hudson better and better, first as a dedicated, deeply committed student, now as a colleague on our Center for Mind-Body Medicine faculty. It's always a joy when he is teaching in our trainings to feel the kindness and wisdom he brings to those we teach, to feel his presence—as knowledgeable, comforting, and dependable as any physician I know. I

Foreword

feel blessed to work with him and learn from him. And I believe, as you read what he has written and walk with Tom Hudson on your own journey—whether it's one of prevention, cancer treatment, or to a deeper experience of life—you will feel the same.

—*Jim Gordon*

Preface

"What causes this?" she asked, referring to her newly diagnosed breast cancer. "No one in my family has ever had it."

"Nobody knows," I answered, wishing I had something more to offer. It was an exchange that had become all too familiar over the years. And each time I was asked, my reply felt emptier than the last.

What was it about this simple question that haunted me? Why did it seem different from the thousands of others I've been asked? Maybe it was the hint of desperation in their voice. Not over what they were facing. People are always more courageous than they think. Most everyone is willing to face what he or she must in a crisis.

No, the despair wasn't over the diagnosis. It was over the lack of anything concrete they could do about it. They wanted information. Something—*anything*—they could do to keep from dying of this disease, or better yet, to keep from getting it in the first place.

Which brings me to an interesting thing about "the question"—*everyone* seemed to be asking it. It wasn't just newly diagnosed women; it was long-term survivors, women considered at high risk, and women with no special risk who asked out of curiosity more than anything else. Everyone wanted to prevent something, whether it was getting breast cancer, having it recur, or dying of it. It was my first revelation that prevention knows no boundaries.

The concept of prevention was not part of my reality at the time. Being a product of traditional medicine, I didn't consider it possible. The survival statistics for breast cancer are spectacularly good compared to many other cancers. We have the finest in modern surgical techniques, the most up-to-date regimens of radiation and chemotherapy, and the best in early detection. But women wanted to know what they could do for themselves beyond that. And when they asked, our words always came up empty. Long before I had ever heard of the term "self-care," it became clear to me that women were interested in doing it.

It was the "What's causing this?" question, and its clearly implied companion, "What can I do about it?" that started me on my search. Surely *somebody* had the answer. Or at least some theories. I needed a small something to give them. A shred of hope. A hand in controlling their own destiny. I was tired of having nothing.

It's been a number of years since those early days of my mammography career. And it's been a long search. One that's taken many twists and turns. Some of what I was looking for I found in my own medical literature, and wondered why I hadn't noticed it before. Much of it I found in the world of "alternative medicine"—a strange place for an M.D. to wander into.

In time, I got a clearer picture of what could be done to prevent breast cancer. Much of it was well documented, some of it was more controversial—but it all made sense. Finally, I had a good handle on what women wanted to hear. I just needed a way to tell them.

After years of accumulating information on what women could do for themselves, both to prevent breast cancer *and* enhance their survival if they already had it, I found that my frustrations had changed. I now had something to say, but no time to say it. The modern practice of radiology allowed time for the question, but no time for an adequate answer. Intellectually speaking, I was all dressed up with nowhere to go.

It was out of this dilemma that I got the idea for a book. The need should have been obvious sooner, I suppose. But my view of the world had to expand before I could recognize it. It's been a long time coming, but now it's here—all the information I wish I'd had years ago in a form you can take in at your leisure.

Journey to Hope is a unique book. It is meant to *be* healing, rather than merely be *about* healing. It is a book to be experienced rather than just read. As much as anything else, *Journey to Hope* is about learning how to think differently. We'll discuss in detail why the medical system looks at breast cancer one way, but you need to see it in quite another.

There will be a lot of information presented, but the information is not the most important part. The power lies in the deeper implications, not the information itself. Put aside any preconceived notions and keep an open mind. Small shifts in perspective change everything.

Take your time. Don't read quickly. Consider. Reflect. The longer you linger in a particular section, the more it will deepen. Read and re-read. This is "taking-a-bubble-bath-with-a-glass-of-wine" kind of reading, not the "take-a-quick-shower-and-head-off-to-work" kind.

Each chapter in *Journey to Hope* builds upon the preceding one. But each can also stand on its own. The first four chapters are introductory in nature, but after that you ca n go anywhere you like. If you have an area of concern or special interest you can go directly to that chapter. Then go wherever your curiosity takes you. Don't worry about missing anything. As you go through the book it will become obvious how interconnected everything is. Each subject

Preface

eventually circles back upon itself.

Each chapter is practical, down-to-earth, and easy to understand. The discussions are meant to be thorough but basic. If you are intellectually curious, there are plenty of explanations of how things work. But don't feel like you need to follow them in detail. They add spice, but they're not the main course.

Most of all, *Journey to Hope* is a book to be enjoyed. You'll learn about breast cancer, the medical system, and more. But you'll also learn a lot about yourself. Breast cancer concerns may have brought you here, but you'll leave with a new way of understanding the world, and your place in it. Nothing could be more valuable.

Introduction

In many ways, this book mirrors my own journey from a purely mechanical view of the human body to a more integrated, mind-body-spirit understanding. There was no grand conversion experience or sudden change of ideology. As I looked deeper into the nature of things, it seemed the only logical course to take. An ongoing series of events led me to think differently not only about breast cancer, but about my profession, and even life itself.

It began with my transition from general radiology into the subspecialty of mammography. In the early 1990s, I was put in charge of the mammography section of our radiology practice in Naples, FL, partly because I liked mammography, and partly because I was the youngest member of the group and nobody else wanted to do it. I gladly accepted the position, though I don't think I had much choice.

I'm quite sure it was relief I saw on my colleagues' faces when someone said, "Why doesn't Tom do Mammo?" Many radiologists don't like reading mammograms. It's more nuanced than looking at an abdominal ultrasound or a chest X-ray. And there's the added difficulty of giving results directly to patients, something many radiologists aren't used to.

Introduction

Who could have known that the seemingly off-the-cuff "Let's let Tom do Mammo" remark would propel me into the forefront of breast imaging, the most emotionally intense subspecialty in all of radiology? Soon I was examining patients, explaining mammogram findings, and gaining my first experience with "the question." As my emotional involvement with the patients deepened, I knew I had to find an answer for them—if one existed.

One of the first things I learned was that the majority of breast cancer cases occur in women with no risk factors. I was shocked. "How can that *be*?" I wondered. "Why do we spend so much time talking about risk factors for breast cancer if most women don't have any?" "And why am I just finding this out now?" I had paid attention in school. Nobody mentioned that.

It was the first time I questioned my medical training, wondering who chose what we were taught, what we weren't—and why. In time I came to understand that the medical point of view is just that—a point of view—influenced by culture, medical tradition, *and* economic concerns. It is a logical point of view, but it is neither infallible nor all-inclusive.

My next major epiphany had to do with food. After trying a whole food concentrate (Juice Plus+®) recommended to me by a friend, I experienced some profound physical changes, including increased energy, faster growth of hair and nails, and smoother skin. It consisted only of powdered fruits and vegetables in a capsule, which was a new concept for me at the time. I only tried it because I trusted my friend. But it rocked my world.

If powdered food in a capsule could make that much difference in how I felt, I wondered what would happen if I actually ate better. So I did, learning much along the way about how profoundly diet affects our health. Again, I found myself asking the question, "Why didn't I learn this in school?"

Introduction

The next life-changing event came through my introduction to the Center for Mind-Body Medicine. It was my wife who first made contact with the Center, attending one of their conferences in hopes of helping her friend Sharron, who was struggling with colon cancer. The conference happened to be right across the street from a medical conference I was attending. I went to the "real" conference, my wife attended the other one, and we compared notes in the evenings.

My conference was routine. But I was quite taken aback by what was going on at hers. Meditation? Imagery? Working with the breath? *That* was supposed to help cancer patients? It sounded like New Age mumbo-jumbo to me. But it was important to my wife—so I listened.

Years later, I now find myself on the faculty of the Center for Mind-Body Medicine, which I suppose makes me a Professor of New Age Mumbo-Jumbo. Yes, I now teach what I once ridiculed—a slice of humble pie if there ever was one.

The final piece of the puzzle was the element of spirituality. I never had trouble with the concept of a Supreme Being. I just had trouble believing such a Being had anything to do with me. I saw God as "up there," me as "down here," and didn't see that one had much to do with the other. The possibility that Spirit was interwoven with everyday life was beyond my understanding.

Awakening to spiritual reality often requires a crisis. For me it happened to be a relationship crisis; for many it's a health crisis. The details of the crisis are not important. What's important is that crisis can lead to a deeper experience of life. Breast cancer—or the fear of it—can be the vehicle that takes you there.

Ultimately, *Journey to Hope* is about rediscovering who we are. On the surface it's a book about breast cancer: how to prevent it, and what to do if you have it. But on a deeper level it's about how to live life fully, come what may—something that cannot be done without understanding the power of the human mind and spiritual reality. When we add these to our everyday awareness, a one-dimensional life becomes a three-dimensional life—with benefits that are astonishing, far-reaching, and immediate. In living on the level of physical reality alone, we've been leaving two-thirds of our assets on the table.

When we embrace our three-dimensional nature, all of life changes. Like Alice stepping through the looking glass, nothing is ever the same. Breast cancer concerns can bring you to the looking glass, but whether you step through or not is up to you. The journey is surprising, at times even disconcerting—but it's worth it. The voyage to self-discovery always is.

1

First, a Word to Men

❦

It may seem unusual to begin a book about breast cancer with a chapter for men, but this is not your usual book. If you're a woman please read along, but this chapter is primarily for the guys. If there is a man in your life, ask him to read it. It's important.

Men can and do get breast cancer, but it's extremely rare. It's not anywhere on our radar screen of personal concerns. We have prostates, after all, and that's enough to worry about. Prostate exams are no fun; we all know that. The biopsies are bloody—and *very* personal. And treatment of prostate cancer often results in impotence. But the specter of prostate cancer comes nowhere close to affecting us like breast cancer affects the lives of women.

The medical system feeds women volumes of information about their breast cancer risk, but almost no information on what they can do about it. This is both fearful and disempowering at the same time. It's like telling women they have a time bomb inside of them. We ask them to come by once a year so we can see if it's gone off, but we never tell them how they can defuse the bomb.

There is nothing for them to do but be herded through the mammography center each year, hopefully told everything is okay, and then repeat the process the following year. They know the odds are in their favor, but they know plenty of others who have gotten unexpected bad news. On some level, every woman lives with the fear that one day she'll walk into the mammography clinic—normal, happy, with lots on her agenda for the rest of the afternoon—and leave on a treadmill toward a cancer diagnosis.

I've often imagined women must feel like a herd of zebra crossing the open plain where the lions live. "There are thousands of us and only a few of them," each zebra thinks to herself, "so I'll probably be okay. But on any given day it *could* be me—and there's nothing I can do about it."

Breast cancer is the most feared disease among women, even though they are *ten times* more likely to die of cardiovascular disease.[1] Treatment involves potential disfigurement, possibly even loss of a breast—one of the primary anchors of a woman's sexuality. Because our culture is so fixated on breasts, there is no way to go through treatment without multiple salvos fired directly at a woman's sexuality, self-image, and self-esteem.

Prostates are safely tucked away, so to speak; hidden from sight. Though prostate cancer is more common, it typically strikes at a more advanced age. Fewer men die of it, and if they do, they rarely leave behind school-age children who were depending on them. Yes, treatment for prostate cancer can result in impotence, a major blow to a man, but with few exceptions the outside parts get to stay intact. Maybe they don't work the way we'd like them to, but at least we get to keep them.

It is often said of men that everything from our houses to our bank accounts is about "mine is bigger than yours," which may be truer than any of us would like to admit. Regardless, it's an outward game played with symbols while the real evidence stays safely tucked away. The truth gets to be my (hopefully not so) little secret.

A woman's sexuality, on the other hand, is on display virtually every hour of every day. Breasts are "right up front" in our society. They're plastered on posters and billboards everywhere. Just because you don't see the anatomic version in public doesn't mean the suggestion isn't there. Most of us are unaware of it on a conscious level, but subconsciously it's impossible not to be affected. The next time you're watching a TV commercial or glancing through a magazine, notice how many prominently featured breasts there are.

This might give you some inkling of how strongly a woman's breasts can be tied to her self-image. The advertising world spends a lot of time and money trying to convince her if she doesn't already think so herself. In this cultural background, what must it be like knowing on any given day—without warning—a lump could pop up, or something could be found on a routine mammogram that could cause her to lose her breast, followed by your interest in her, followed by her life? She knows it probably isn't going to happen. But for any woman, it could happen tomorrow. And for a certain number it does.

Many women go to the mammography center together every year, often making a day of it by going to lunch afterwards. But if you think your wife gets together with a close friend or relative once a year for a fun outing to do "lunch and a mammogram," you're wrong. In case you hadn't noticed, women don't pick casual friends to get their mammogram with. They pick those they know will be there for them if they get bad news. It's not about the lunch. They can do lunch any day.

What do they talk about during their time together? The usual: the food, everyday life, and maybe a little about us. But the deeper question they're asking each other is unspoken: "If I get bad news today, will you be there for me?" And merely by going, their mutually unspoken reply is, "Yes, I will." They're sharing much more than lunch and a mutual appointment; they're sharing their fear, their courage—and their commitment to each other. It's beautiful. And it's powerful. Except on the battlefield, it's a bond few men understand.

This is the world a woman inhabits, and though as men we have our own unique challenges, we have nothing like this. I belabor the point because it's important to understand that you don't really understand. Luckily, compassion doesn't require us to have the same experience as someone else. It only asks us to listen and to care. If you do these, your woman will consider you an indispensable part of the emotional team. The benefits for you both are enormous.

One of the themes you'll notice as you go through this book is how interconnected we all are. Male, female, old, young, healthy, or sick—the differences are superficial. Underneath we're all the same. Our interconnection is especially strong in our most intimate relationships. On some level, whatever affects her also affects you and vice-versa. And the effects aren't just relational—they're physical. Wound healing, for example, can be delayed by up to 24 hours after a marital argument, a clear indication of a suppressed immune system.[2] The same immune system that protects against cancer.

Considering this, one of the first things a woman needs to do if she's serious about decreasing her risk of breast cancer is to deal with her relational stress. If she's a survivor or currently going through treatment the stakes are even higher. Sometimes major change is needed. Sometimes it just requires an honest look at an already good relationship to see where it can be improved. Either way, this involves you.

Don't worry—perfection is not required. All relationships are a mixture of good days and bad. As long as the overall health of a relationship is good, a few bad days here and there don't matter. But if the overall pattern is one of underlying stress, a relationship can degrade our health as fast, or faster, as anything else.

No matter what your partner is wrestling with, don't underestimate how much you can help simply by being understanding and supportive. *You* are as much the medicine as any medicine she may be getting. And you are a large piece of the cancer prevention puzzle as well. We'll discuss this in more detail in the chapter on relationships, but hearing it up front will help you understand how important it is.

Whether you're a man or a woman, if you embark on this journey, you will be making changes in your life that will enhance your health and well-being immensely. In doing so, you may wake up tomorrow and find that you're not the same person you were yesterday. This is a wonderful thing, because as humans we're happiest and healthiest when we're growing emotionally and spiritually.

It's even more wonderful if the one we love takes the journey with us. We bump into each other a lot less when we're headed in the same direction. So don't let your woman go it alone. Read the book. Be with her in this. Put your novels aside for a month and share this experience with her. Do it wholeheartedly. Your efforts will be richly rewarded.

Your support will benefit her immensely, but there's a lot in it for you, too. You'll gain a deeper understanding of what women go through, and you'll learn a lot about yourself in the process. Yes, this is a book about breast cancer, but it's really about the human experience, and how best to live it. It's a book for everyone—men, women, cancer survivors, and those who will never be touched by cancer. Share the experience with the one you love. It may be one of the best things you ever did.

2

What's My Risk?

❧

"How likely am I to get breast cancer?" That's what everyone wants to know. Even if you're a survivor or have been recently diagnosed, it's just a different form of the same question: "What are my chances?" As with most things in life, it's not as simple as it seems.

The pat answer is 1 in 8. At the present time, roughly 1 in 8 women in the U.S. will develop breast cancer at some point in their life. The 1 in 8 statistic is simple, recognizable, and quite correct. It reflects how common breast cancer is in this country. It has become a slogan, used to encourage women to get their yearly mammogram in hopes of catching the disease early when it's at a more treatable stage. But like any statistic, 1 in 8 can be misleading.

If you're at the hair salon and happen to notice seven other women there it's easy to think one of you may have breast cancer and doesn't know it yet. But that isn't what 1 in 8 means. The 1 in 8 statistic represents a woman's lifetime risk of developing breast cancer to age ninety.[1] If you're not ninety years old, the number doesn't apply to you.

Breast cancer risk is age-related. The younger you are the less common it is. But age is only one of many factors that affect your risk. Let's take a look at some of the others:[2,3]

Chapter Two

Gender: Simply being female is the largest risk factor for breast cancer. It's exceedingly rare in males. Men are one hundred times less likely to get breast cancer than women.

Race: White, non-Hispanic women have the highest incidence of breast cancer in the U.S., while Korean American women have the lowest. African American women have the highest incidence between the ages of forty and fifty, and the highest death rate at any age. Chinese American women have the lowest death rate.

Age: Your risk of developing breast cancer increases with age. Breast cancer risk stated as an age-related number gives you much better information than the 1 in 8 statistic. If your age is:

30-39 your risk is 1 in 233
40-49 your risk is 1 in 69
50-59 your risk is 1 in 42
60-69 your risk is 1 in 29

For each age range, these numbers represent your risk of being diagnosed with breast cancer in the next ten years. The 1 in 8 statistic is a reflection of the country at large. The age related numbers have a lot more to do with you.

Reproductive/hormonal factors: The earlier in life you begin menstruating and the later you reach menopause the greater your risk of breast cancer.[4] The later in life you have children the greater the risk. Breastfeeding decreases your risk.[5] You are at a higher risk if you've never had children. All of these factors are thought to be due to estrogenic effects.[6,7] Most breast cancers are related to high levels of circulating estrogen. American women have some of the highest estrogen levels in the world, for reasons we'll discuss later.

Family history: If other family members have been diagnosed with breast cancer it increases the likelihood you will develop it as well. This is one of the strongest risk factors.[8] The more members of your family that have been diagnosed, and the closer they are in relation to you, the greater your risk. Your risk would be greater, for instance, if your mother and sister had breast cancer than if it were two cousins or aunts.

Genetic breast cancer: Breast cancer that occurs in women with a family history is not considered true "genetic" breast cancer. Only cases occurring in women who are carriers of the BRCA1 or BRCA2 gene mutations are considered genetic. This is the strongest risk factor of all. Women with these gene mutations have up to five times the risk of the average woman.[9] Luckily, genetic breast cancer is uncommon, representing only five to ten percent of all cases.

Risk Models

A little known fact about breast cancer risk is that the myriad risk factors are not necessarily additive.[10] If your increased risk is estimated to be ten percent due to factor A, thirty percent due to factor B, and twenty percent due to factor C, you don't necessarily have a sixty percent increased risk. There have been thousands of studies on the subject of breast cancer risk, but few have dealt with combinations of risk factors.

No woman has only one risk factor. Every woman has some factors that increase her risk and some that decrease it. Nobody knows how they all fit together. Just a glance at the factors we've discussed so far will give you an idea of how impossibly complex an overall risk assessment can be.

There are mathematical models that consider combinations of risk factors but they can be misleading. The accuracy of any particular model will be limited by the number of risk factors that model takes into account. The models aren't all the same.[11,12] It's not at all uncommon to be considered high risk by one model and average risk by another. Risk assessment is not an exact science by any means.

A major weakness with current risk assessment models is that you have no control over any of the risk factors included in the calculations. Your reproductive history is mostly set by the time you're old enough to begin having mammograms. You have no control over when you begin to menstruate or when you stop. Your age is your age, your gender is your gender, and most especially—your family is your family.

Family history is by far he most heavily weighted factor in all of the risk assessment models. This fits nicely with the medical paradigm of genetic determinism, which holds that cancer forms from "bad genes." From this viewpoint it makes perfect sense that you can't do anything about your breast cancer risk because your risk is largely inherited.

The problem with any family history-based risk model is that only a minority of cases actually fit the model. In fact, 75 percent of all breast cancer occurs in women with *no known risk factor*.[13] This is a startling statistic. Clearly, we have to begin thinking differently about this disease. The current models of breast cancer risk raise more questions than they answer.

Other Risk Factors

There have been more research studies done on the subject of breast cancer than any other type of cancer.[14] Many studies have identified risk factors other than those the traditional medical model focuses on. Some of the research evidence for these is strong. Some is not. The compelling reason to take a look at them is that they include things you can actually do something about. They are "modifiable" risk factors.

High-Fat Diet: This was one of the first modifiable risk factors to become part of the larger medical discussion. Research studies are conflicting for reasons we'll discuss later, but many studies show that women who consume a large percentage of their calories as fat have a higher incidence of breast cancer than those who do not.

Obesity/Level of Physical Activity: Your breast cancer risk increases in proportion to how overweight you are. Obese women have a sixty percent greater risk than women of normal weight.[15] This effect is limited to post-menopausal women for reasons we will discuss in chapter five. Physical activity also plays a role. Women who get an adequate amount of exercise cut their risk by half or more.[16,17]

Alcohol: For each drink you have per day, your risk of developing breast cancer goes up eleven percent.[18] If you have two drinks per day, your risk is twenty-two percent higher. For three drinks, it's thirty-three percent.

Stress: Some studies show an increased incidence of breast cancer in women who describe themselves as chronically stressed.[19] Women who have experienced recent traumatic life events such as divorce or the death of a loved one may also be at increased risk.[20] The elevated risk seems to be based on how well women cope with these stressful events rather than the events themselves.[21]

The Bigger Picture

The above, only a partial list, makes a compelling case that breast cancer is more than a genetic disease. Not only is the environment a factor, but our personal choices are as well. Despite this, the medical discussion remains focused on age and family history as the most important risk factors. A closer look will further dispel the notion that breast cancer is predominantly an inherited disease.

Cancer is well known to occur more commonly in some geographic areas than others.[22] Breast cancer is rare in third world nations. It is much more common in industrialized countries. Asia has a far lower incidence of breast cancer than the U.S. The incidence in Western Europe is similar to ours.

This might be attributed to genetic differences except for immigration studies showing that risk increases in women who leave countries with a low incidence of breast cancer and move to a country with a high incidence.[23] After a generation or two, immigrants take on the same breast cancer risk of the country they immigrate to—even if they don't intermarry.[24,25]

Studies of adopted children lead to the same conclusion. Girls who are adopted at a young age take on the breast cancer risk of their adopted family, not their family of origin. The environment they grow up in is more important than the genes they carry.[26]

Studies of identical twins point to the same thing. From a strictly genetic standpoint, if a twin is diagnosed with breast cancer, the other twin should be doomed to get it too. But most of them don't. Only twenty-five percent of breast cancer risk in identical twins is due to genetic factors.[27]

The 1 in 8 statistic itself is a strong argument against heredity being the overriding factor in breast cancer risk. In the 1940s the number was 1 in 22 and has been steadily rising ever since. What could cause such a dramatic rise in the breast cancer rate in just a few generations? The gene pool hasn't changed.

Any one of these facts would be enough to cast serious doubt on the genetic determinism argument. Taken together they make this point of view completely untenable. Attributing all your risk to family history and reproductive factors doesn't make sense when it can't explain three-quarters of the cases. Even those cases attributable to family history may not be due to inheritance alone. Members of the same family live in the same place, eat the same food, are exposed to the same environmental toxins, and tend to have the same emotional patterns. How many of the family history cases might be attributable to these factors rather than heredity?

Epigenetics

The new science of epigenetics makes it clear we're asking the wrong question when we debate how much of breast cancer risk is due to the environment and how much is due to heredity. It isn't one or the other; it's both. The development of cancer has to do with the *interaction* between your genes and the environment, not either one alone. Epigenetics is the study of this interaction.

Genetic determinism, the prevailing view of Western science, maintains that the gene is everything. Our genes determine the color of our hair, our height, our IQ, and everything about us, including our susceptibility to disease. Cancer, like many diseases, tends to run in families. It's assumed we simply inherit the tendency to get it from our parents. From this perspective, your breast cancer risk was largely set the day you were born.

Breast cancer in women with no family history is assumed to occur when normal genes spontaneously mutate. Or in other words, when perfectly good genes go bad. Environmental factors are acknowledged to play a role only in special cases.

Recent research, however, shows genetic determinism to be too simplistic. To date, the human genome project has identified between 30,000 and 45,000 genes, far fewer than expected. There are not nearly enough genes to encode for all known human traits. We have only slightly more genes than the common earthworm, and fewer than rice.[28] Clearly there is much we don't understand.

In some cases we carry a gene for a certain trait, yet the trait is not expressed. The gene exists in our DNA, but by looking at the individual one sees no evidence of it. Research has shown that each gene has a corresponding "mark," which is cellular material sitting directly on top of the gene that controls its expression—effectively turning it "on" and "off." Taken together, these marks constitute an entire *epi*genome that controls how our genes function (*epi-* is the Greek prefix for *above*).

Genes themselves are not "intelligent." They can only do what they're programmed to do. They are a code for the basic infrastructure, nothing more. Our genes are a blueprint—not the determining factor of everything in our lives. The nucleus, which contains all the genetic material, is *not* the brain of the cell; it's the reproductive organ.

Epigenetic marks turn our genes on and off depending on the needs of the organism, but even they don't function independently. They need a brain to tell them what to do. In the world of the cell, this role is filled by the cell membrane.[29] The cell membrane communicates with the epigenome by way of messenger molecules telling it exactly what's needed.

Only the cell membrane can know what's needed because it alone is in contact with the outside world. It decides what gets in, what gets out, and tells the genetic material what to make, how much, and when. It is the perceiver and the chooser—a large part of the body's innate intelligence.

How does the cell membrane perceive the environment and know the proper course to take in perfect concert with trillions of its counterparts? Is the intricate network of our cell membranes part and parcel of a higher intelligence? This is, and always will be, a mystery. There's nothing in the physical structure itself that can give us an answer.

However it works, it's clear our body has an intelligence all its own, functioning below the level of our everyday awareness. This intelligence interacts with the environment on a moment-to-moment basis, influencing how our genes function.

Animal models have proven that the environment directly affects gene expression. Mice raised in an enriched environment show increased cortical thickness in their brains at autopsy.[30] MRI brain scans show a similar effect in people who meditate regularly, presumably through the same mechanism—certain genes are "turned on," producing more brain tissue in response to a healthy interaction with the environment.[31]

The implications in terms of cancer are profound. If genes respond to a healthy environment by producing healthy cells, could they respond to an unhealthy environment by producing unhealthy cells? Increased cortical thickness is due to controlled production of normal brain cells. Cancer is uncontrolled production of abnormal cells. If the environment can stimulate one, surely it is capable of the other.

Not only can the environment affect how our genes behave in a single lifetime, the effects can also be passed on to the next generation.[32] Dietary changes and stressful events experienced by one generation have been shown to affect gene expression in the next.[33,34] This means that stressful events and environmental exposures experienced by your parents can affect how *your* genes function.

Everything we inherit does not necessarily involve the unchangeable genetic code. Genes that were turned on in one generation can be turned off in the next—if you respond to the environment differently than your parents did. How much could this affect your breast cancer risk? No one knows. But epigenetics provides a mechanism for what studies on immigrants, twins, and adopted children have already told us: breast cancer risk is something that can be altered.

Genetic determinism has been the prevailing view of Western science since Watson and Crick discovered the double helix in 1953. Even though more recent data show this view to be outdated, traditional thinking on the matter has changed little. It is important to understand that your breast cancer risk is communicated to you by a medical community that remains deeply mired in this paradigm.

In terms of cancer risk, genetic determinism tells us that little we do matters. But a more updated version of genetics tells us that *everything* we do matters. Which of these you believe makes a world of difference. One leads to passive indifference; the other to engaged action. It can mean the difference between despair and hope. And for some—life and death.

Epigenetics even gives us a more updated definition of the environment. From a cellular perspective everything outside the cell membrane is the "environment," even if a particular cell membrane lies deep within the body. Everything we see, hear, touch, taste, and smell is perceived through a cell membrane of some kind.

What's My Risk?

In terms of cancer, it is the cellular environment that matters because cancer is a process that begins in a single cell. To a cell there is no difference between toxic chemicals and toxic emotions. They both expose cell membranes to a "hostile environment," information that is immediately communicated to your DNA. How does the DNA respond? It depends. Is the response enough to cause cancer? Many believe the answer is yes.

Conventional medical wisdom dismisses dietary, psychological, and emotional factors in breast cancer risk as unscientific because they're difficult to get a handle on. While this may be true, these factors have more of a scientific basis than many realize. There's a lot of evidence showing that what you eat, what you think, and how you feel affects your risk of disease. In his book, *Biology of Belief*, cell biologist Bruce Lipton makes a compelling case that even what you *believe* affects your risk—something spiritual teachers have been telling us for millennia.[35] This type of thinking is not part of the traditional medical perspective, but many feel it should be.

Breast Cancer Prevention

Understanding that it's the interaction between our genes and the environment that causes cancer is empowering. Finally, here's something you have some control over. Remembering that negative emotions and chronic stress are also environmental toxins from a cellular perspective places even more of the equation within your grasp. Can breast cancer be prevented? The evidence strongly suggests it can. This is good news, but a word of caution is in order.

If a woman never gets breast cancer, it's impossible to know whether some action she took prevented it or if she would have never gotten it in the first place. And of the women who do get cancer, there's no way to know if it could have been prevented or not. There's nothing about the cancer itself that can tell us one way or the other. Prevention can be statistically proven in large groups of women, but can never be proven in an individual.

If we could pin down a primary cause for breast cancer it would be easy, but there's no "smoking gun" for breast cancer like cigarette smoking is for lung cancer. There are dozens of factors that correlate with a high breast cancer incidence, but correlation is very different than causation. A woman with breast cancer could point to any number of factors that might have "caused" her cancer. But for any of these, there are more women with the same risk factor that don't get breast cancer than do.

Human interaction with the environment is complex. Not everyone who is exposed to a cancer-causing substance gets cancer. Cancer is very much a "seed and the soil" process, with cancer-causing substances from the environment being the seed, and our bodies the soil.

From this standpoint prevention is simple: avoid as many bad seeds as you can, including the self-inflicted ones, and do everything in your power to enhance your soil. The state of your general health and the integrity of your immune system are your strongest defenses against cancer.

Doing Everything Right

The possibility of preventing cancer would seem to be good news for everyone, but it can be disconcerting for some. For women who have already been diagnosed, dealing with the fact their cancer might have been prevented can be a challenge. These women fall into two categories: those who actively took steps to prevent breast cancer but got it anyway, and those who didn't take preventive measures but later learned if they had, things might have been different.

Women in the first group tend to feel angry. From their perspective they "did everything right," which to most means eating a healthy diet and getting plenty of exercise. There's a sense of betrayal when they do these things and get breast cancer anyway. Women in the second group tend to blame themselves. "If breast cancer is preventable and I got it, on some level it must be my fault," is how the thinking goes.

For both groups, the complexities of breast cancer risk assessment are a blessing. No matter what you do, you *can't* do everything right. It's too complex for that. Diet and exercise are important, but they're only part of a much larger picture. Chronic stress and unhealthy emotional patterns may also play a role in your risk. And there are many more unknowns. It's impossible to avoid every known cancer-causing substance, and even if you did there are more floating around that haven't been identified yet.

The complexities involved make it clear there is no basis for beating yourself up over what might have been. No matter what you did or didn't do, you can never know if it would have made any difference. There's no sense crying over spilled milk you can't be sure you even spilled.

The "I did everything right" group and the "I should have done better" group are actually opposite sides of the same coin, revealing a thinking pattern indicative of the culture at large. Western thinking is largely "dualistic." It sees things in terms of black and white, all or none, and either/or.

Dualistic thinking says, "If I do this or don't do that, I can avoid an unpleasant outcome 100 percent of the time." It's always looking for simple answers, guarantees, and magic bullets. It is a comforting thought pattern because it reduces everything down to simple terms. But the comfort gives way to disappointment when we find out the issues weren't as simple as we thought.

Decreasing Your Risk

Despite the uncertainties, breast cancer prevention is an established fact, and it's something you should pursue. Because the term prevention can lead to false expectations, however, I prefer to use the phrase "decreasing your risk" instead. The term prevention, though technically true, is a little too black and white. It overpromises—and occasionally underdelivers.

"Decreasing your risk," on the other hand, always delivers what it promises—to improve your chances. Inherent in the phrase is the lack of a guarantee. No matter what you do or how well you do it, your risk of breast cancer will never be zero. Life itself is a risky proposition. Understanding this and making peace with it will allow you to properly interpret all the information that follows.

Don't think in terms of doing everything right. Think in terms of doing as much for yourself as you can, realizing you'll never do it perfectly. And if you're a survivor, don't waste time looking back wondering "What if." You will learn things in this book you could have put to good use years ago, but that's true for any area of life. Let the new information empower you to build a healthier future, not drag you back to a past you're powerless to change.

For those women who take the steps outlined in this book, some will not get breast cancer that would have otherwise. I just can't promise that will be you. But taking the steps has a value beyond the question of breast cancer. Taken together, they will enhance your experience of life. Take the steps. Do the work. Trust the process. It will take you where you want to go. ❧

3

The New Medicine

This book is about taking charge of your own health, a concept known as self-care. It represents a new way of thinking about health care—one that is centered on you, not the medical system. Self-care is the centerpiece of what has been called the New Medicine. To understand why this is a new way of thinking about healthcare, you will first have to understand current medical thinking. This requires a few words about systems and paradigms.

Systems and Paradigms

A system is a group of interacting, interrelated, or interdependent elements forming a complex whole. Systems have personalities, tendencies, and certain ways of thinking, just like a person. In essence, a system can be thought of as a person without a body. The word "corporation" comes from the Latin word *corpus*, which means body.

The world is full of systems. There is a medical system, an insurance system, and a financial system. There are religious systems and systems of government. Even businesses and families can be considered systems.

Chapter Three

Every system has its unique way of seeing the world, and everyone within the system is subject to that particular pattern of thinking. It's like an invisible brain that influences everyone in the system. Once someone becomes part of a system, their point of view tends to fall in line with the system's point of view, no matter what they thought before. This well-known phenomenon has been referred to as "groupthink." The overall pattern of thinking is called a paradigm.

A paradigm is a set of shared assumptions regarding what works or what is true. Wikipedia refers to a paradigm as the box in "thinking outside the box." A paradigm is similar to a point of view or a perspective, only more pervasive. It is a way of seeing the world. It affects how you interpret everything.

By definition, paradigms are limiting. To someone stuck in a paradigm, the world consists only of the box. The problem is, the world is bigger than that. The box itself also skews the interpretation of reality. Those inside the box do not perceive events in the same way as those outside it. What seems self-evident to someone within a system may make no sense at all to anyone else.

This is why it sometimes "makes sense" for the government to pay $75 for a hammer and $200 for a toilet seat, even though this sounds ridiculous to the rest of us. Many people at multiple levels have to sign off on such purchases, and it's important to understand they are just like you and me.

When Portuguese explorer Ferdinand Magellan landed on an island in the New World, the natives came out to shore to meet him. In response to their obvious curiosity, he pointed to his ships anchored offshore. Even though the ships were in plain view, the natives couldn't see them. Because they had no frame of reference for tall ships, the natives were unable to see what was in plain sight. They were eventually able to see the ships, but only after the tribal shaman came and instructed them to look with their peripheral vision.

Whether the story is true or apocryphal, it shows us what paradigms are at its core—a type of blindness; a symptom of limited perspective. The shaman had no problem seeing the ships even though he had never seen such a sight before either. Presumably this was due to his broader perspective as the spiritual leader of the tribe.

A broader perspective is the antidote to limiting paradigms. In effect, it breaks down the walls of the box, allowing us to see what we previously could not. Our box defines the limits of our *perception* of reality, but it doesn't define reality. What goes on outside of our awareness affects us whether we are aware of it or not. Expanding our perspective puts us more in tune with how things really are—not just how we *think* they are.

Like that of any individual, the medical point of view is limited. Knowing what those limitations are is enormously helpful. Understanding how the system "thinks" will help you negotiate your way more peacefully, properly interpret any advice you are given, and help you make better decisions. It will help you know when to go with the flow, and when to swim against the current.

The Current Biomedical Model

We have already discussed part of the medical paradigm in terms of breast cancer—genetic determinism. The paradigm effect explains why the medical system doggedly holds to a family history-based model of breast cancer risk, even though scientific evidence indicates otherwise.

This is exasperating to those who think differently, but perfectly logical to those who hold the same point of view. Remember, a paradigm is a shared set of assumptions regarding what is true. It doesn't have to actually *be* true. To those who share the assumptions, it *is* true. And they are unable to see it differently, despite evidence to the contrary.

Drugs and surgery are two additional pieces of the current medical paradigm. Taken together they form the centerpiece of the system (fig. 1). The majority of all visits to the doctor result in a prescription. And when medication is no longer effective, surgery is the next logical step.

Some people prefer to go to "alternative" medical practitioners: acupuncturists, chiropractors, energy healers, and so on, but they mostly go on their own. They are rarely referred by a medical doctor. They either go because they believe in that system of care, or because they are dissatisfied with the conventional medical system. Sometimes both.[1] There is a wide gulf between the two systems, which patients have to bridge on their own.

In the current medical model, there is virtually no communication between conventional and alternative practitioners. Most physicians don't see the need. In the vast majority of medical schools, there is no nutritional education, no discussion of natural remedies, and no exposure to alternative health fields—not even an overview of what they do.

The current model is supported by governmental and insurance systems that reimburse for traditional medical therapies, but not for alternative therapies. By and large, when someone mentions the healthcare system, they mean pharmaceutical-based conventional medicine. Alternative therapies are not considered part of the system.

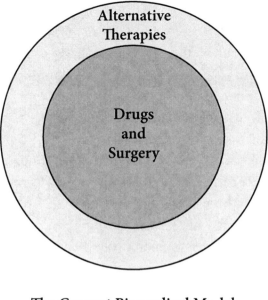

The Current Biomedical Model
(fig. 1)

(with permission. James S. Gordon, M.D., Center for Mind-Body Medicine)

How well is this working? Not as well as those within the system would like to think. Pharmaceuticals are overused and the side effects can be dangerous. The U.S. consumes nearly fifty percent of the world's supply of pharmaceuticals despite having only five percent of the world's population.[2] The number of those addicted to prescription medication has surpassed the number addicted to illegal drugs, and more people die annually from prescription drug overdose than overdose of illegal drugs.[3,4] Over 100,000 deaths in the U.S. occur each year from properly prescribed medication, and another 80,000 from improperly prescribed medication.[5]

Pharmaceuticals are strong medicine. They're high reward—but also high risk. They are the backbone of the medical system,

Chapter Three

but they're not making us any healthier. In the World Health Organization's most recent healthcare rankings, the United States was 37th overall out of the 39 industrialized nations. We were a dismal 72nd out of 191 in health of the population—even though we ranked number one in per capita health spending.[6,7]

Fortunately, it's not all bad news. The U.S. was ranked number one in responsiveness of its healthcare system. Responsiveness is based on many factors, but it roughly corresponds to what most would call "acute care." What it basically means is if you are hit by a bus or collapse at the grocery store with a heart attack, your chances of surviving are better here than anywhere in the world. And pharmaceuticals will likely play a major role in saving your life.

Modern medicine, like everything in life, is a double-edged sword. It does some things incredibly well and other things poorly. When it comes to acute care, we're the best in the world. When it comes to the prevention and treatment of chronic disease, we don't do nearly as well. In the acute setting, pharmaceuticals can save your life. In the setting of chronic disease, they tend to mask symptoms without addressing the root cause of the disease. They make us feel better, but they don't make our underlying problem go away.

The landscape is changing in some areas. When it comes to heart disease, prevention has become mainstream. Any cardiologist or family practitioner will tell you how important diet and lifestyle are in preventing a heart attack or stroke. The importance of diet and lifestyle in cancer prevention, however, remains largely unrecognized. The role of nutrition, stress reduction, and psychological factors in cancer risk is firmly established in the alternative world. It's mostly not on the radar screen in the conventional world.

The New Medicine

The current medical model is out of balance in many ways. Having drugs and surgery, the riskiest modalities, as the centerpiece is the first sign something is amiss. Another sign is that the health-care system as we know it is misnamed. It is a *disease*-care system, not a true healthcare system. As physicians, we study disease. We learn how to detect it early and how to treat it. Even a yearly physical is a mini-diagnostic session looking for potential problems.

There's nothing wrong with that. People get injured and they get sick. And they need someone with the technology and expertise to help them when they do. It's nice to have big guns available when they're needed, and drugs and surgery are big guns.

Big guns can cause collateral damage, however, which is why it's good to save them until they're needed. This is what a more comprehensive medical model (fig. 2) is all about—saving them until they're needed. Nobody wants to do away with medicine as we know it. The New Medicine doesn't throw out the old; it just adds the missing pieces. And some perspective.

Self-care is the centerpiece of the New Medicine and the focus of this book. It only makes sense to start with what you can do for yourself. It's also logical to access practitioners who can help maintain your health and deal with small problems before they become big ones. This is what alternative practices do.

These practices are referred to as "CAM" (complementary/alternative medicine) in the new medical model to underscore the fact that it needn't be either/or in terms of alternative vs. conventional medicine. Many CAM therapies enhance conventional medical treatments. In an ideal world they would be used together.

Conventional medicine may consider alternative practices unscientific, but there are over 450,000 published articles on these practices listed in the NCCAM (National Center for Complementary and Alternative Medicine) database on PubMed.[8] Physicians may see them as peripheral, but increasing numbers of people do not. Nearly seventy percent of cancer patients visit alternative practitioners and eighty percent say they would like more information.[9] More and more people are going, but few of them tell their doctors about it—a fact that reflects poorly on doctors, not patients.

Many physicians are developing "integrative" practices, meaning they offer CAM treatments in addition to traditional medical therapies. Again, this only makes sense. Conventional medicine focuses on treating disease. Alternative medicine focuses on healing the whole person, which sometimes results in spontaneous regression of disease. The two are not mutually exclusive.

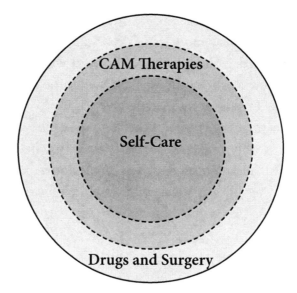

The New Medicine
(fig. 2)

(with permission. James S. Gordon, M.D., Center for Mind-Body Medicine)

In the new model, the lines between self-care, CAM practitioners, and conventional medicine are blurred. Just because you're making use of one doesn't preclude you from accessing the others at the same time. Healing belongs to the human family. It can't be divided any more than the sea or the sky. Whatever works, works. None of it is anybody's property. In the New Medicine, conventional and alternative practitioners actually talk to each other. It is fully integrated. There aren't separate systems; only one "comprehensive" healthcare system.

The Great Divide

The current gulf between conventional and alternative medicine can be both astonishing and humorous at the same time. A friend of mine recently called a local medical office and asked if they practiced complementary medicine. She was put on hold while the receptionist went to get an answer for her. When the receptionist came back on the line, she told my friend, "No, we don't do any 'complimentary' medicine. We charge for everything."

To those familiar with the alternative world, it sounds like a comedy routine. But considering the state of medical education and the stranglehold the pharmaceutical industry has on the medical paradigm, there's no reason to *expect* a typical medical office to know anything about complementary medicine.

Going from one system to the other is like crossing the border into a different country. Each system has its own language, its own worldview, and attracts different types of people. There is value in both systems, but too few practitioners are willing to cross the border. Many in conventional medicine don't even know there's a border to cross.

If you're going to access the conventional medical system—whether for a routine mammogram, end-stage cancer treatment, or anything in between—it's enormously helpful to know what you can expect from the system and what you cannot. Unless you go to an integrative medical practice, they're unlikely to know much about alternative or complementary modalities, and unlikely to refer you to anyone who does.

Considering this "great divide," it should come as no surprise that mainstream medicine's concept of breast cancer prevention is heavily slanted toward drugs and surgery. If you visit the American Cancer Society website and search for breast cancer prevention, you'll find detailed discussions on chemoprevention (Tamoxifen and related drugs) and surgical prevention (prophylactic mastectomy), but little else.[10] This is a reflection of the conventional medical point of view. It's just how the system sees things.

A current advertisement on the WebMD website sums up the medical viewpoint on prevention: "Wouldn't it be amazing if women at high risk for breast cancer could pop a pill?"[11] Understand, there's nothing wrong with the pill. The only thing wrong is emphasizing the pill without including information on how to decrease your risk *without* the pill. Or what you can do to enhance the pill's effectiveness if you decide to take it.

To be fair, a few of the modifiable risk factors are mentioned on these sites, but the mention is so brief and so understated compared to the more detailed discussions on Tamoxifen and prophylactic mastectomy, one is left with the impression they're not very important. But they're enormously important.

Yes, some women will need to know about Tamoxifen, but every woman needs to know what she can do to decrease her breast cancer risk without the side effects of drugs, and while keeping her breasts if she chooses. It makes sense to include Tamoxifen and prophylactic mastectomy in the discussion; it just doesn't make sense to start there. They should be the last resort, not considered the only resort. There *are* other options.

Women who exercise more than four hours a week, for instance, cut their breast cancer risk in half.[12] Adequate exercise can reduce mortality in breast cancer patients by the same amount.[13] Women who have exercised throughout their lifetime decrease their risk even more.[14] Exercise increases immunity, improves mood, reduces symptoms, and increases longevity. There is no medical therapy that can say the same. On top of that, it's something you can do for yourself, as opposed to something we have to do for you.

This is potentially life-saving information. It is duly noted by the medical community, but not emphasized. It's posted on bulletin boards, but not shouted from the rooftops. And it's not just about exercise. Other lifestyle changes can decrease your risk by just as much. The information is available, but the medical paradigm has not shifted enough to see its importance.

Paradigm Shifts

Thomas Kuhn coined the term "paradigm shift" in his influential book, *The Structure of Scientific Revolutions* (1962). Simply put, if a paradigm is a set of shared assumptions, a paradigm shift is a change in the basic assumptions. It is a change in thinking from an accepted point of view to a new one, necessitated when new scientific discoveries reveal anomalies in the current paradigm.

The fact that three-quarters of breast cancer cases don't fit the current paradigm is an anomaly of gigantic proportions, telling us that a paradigm shift is long overdue. It's not surprising, however, that one has not yet occurred.

System paradigms can and do change, but progress is typically slow, even ponderous. Broad-based system change usually comes decades after enough new information surfaces to warrant it. No one likes change—systems least of all. Paradigm shifts are about expanding the walls of the box. The problem is, those walls represent our comfort zone, and moving them can be uncomfortable. Our individual walls are rigid. System walls are monolithic.

The concept of paradigms explains why some physicians find the WHO healthcare rankings and the information on pharmaceutical-related deaths challenging. Most are unaware of it, and many refuse to believe it even after they hear it. Yet it is well documented by reputable sources.

The WHO is an independent, well-respected institution without an axe to grind. The information on drug-related deaths comes from an article written by physicians and published in the Journal of the American Medical Association (JAMA). As physicians, if it makes us uncomfortable, it's a good sign. It means the walls of the box are beginning to bend.

The Bigger Picture

The WHO rankings and pharmaceutical statistics may seem to be aimed directly at the medical system, but they're not. The medical system doesn't exist in a vacuum. Like any system, it is a reflection of the culture at large. Do doctors prescribe too much medication when safer techniques are available? Advocates of the New Medicine would say yes. But this is only part of a much larger picture.

Many patients come to the doctor's office demanding medication, and doctors are often afraid not to prescribe it because of malpractice concerns. Pharmaceutical companies spend billions each year on television advertising. If we watch TV, we are indoctrinated from a young age to believe that pharmaceuticals are the way to go.

The New Medicine

The problem is multi-faceted, but it boils down to a cultural bias toward relying on a pill to fix whatever ails us, absolving us of the responsibility to take care of ourselves. We expect to live however we want and look to the medical system to bail us out when the boat starts to sink. It's not that we're irresponsible; it's the cultural paradigm. We're taught to believe that the pharmaceutical-based medical system is our savior. In some cases it is. In most cases it's not.

There is an inherent contradiction to expecting a pill to cure a lifestyle disease. The WHO rankings make it painfully clear that it's never going to work. It's comforting to think the medical system will take care of everything for us, but the system isn't designed to do that. The healthcare system can help when things go wrong, but despite its name, it can't make us healthy—only we can do that.

It is unwise to give the power over your health away to the healthcare system. Medical advice is just that—advice. Consider it, but take into account the paradigm out of which the advice comes— and then do what you think best. Gone are the days of "patient compliance," where your doctor tells you what to do and you're considered a bad patient if you don't do it.

In the new medical paradigm, the concept of compliance is replaced by *collaboration*, which reflects the healing relationship between doctor and patient. As physicians, we're here to serve, to advise, and to help you make informed decisions. The decision itself is up to you. When you ask your physician about breast cancer prevention and he or she talks about pills and scalpels, you can be assured of their expertise. Just remember there is another point of view.

Chapter Three

Rising Tide

When will the New Medicine be here? Change is already underway. The mindset of the population is slowly shifting away from the traditional healthcare paradigm to one that's more integrative in nature. As the mindset of the population shifts, systems are swept along with it. The number of organic farms is increasing, restaurants are offering healthier food choices, visits to alternative practitioners are increasing, and there is increased interest in disease prevention.

Physicians who integrate their practices do quite well, and are typically healthier and happier than their more conventional colleagues. Susan Blum, M.D., M.P.H., who recently opened an integrative health center in Rye Brook, N.Y., says of her work, "I feel like I won the lottery every day." Such statements are unheard of in conventional medical practice.

The changing medical landscape brings the focus of your health back to you. This puts the question of breast cancer prevention, with the caveats we discussed in the last chapter, squarely in your lap. When will the New Medicine be here? In many ways it's already here. It's just waiting for us to notice. ❧

4

Self-Care

❧

If ever there was a concept whose time has come, it is self-care. It is the heart of the New Medicine, and makes sense on so many levels. In maintaining your health, it's always best to start with the easiest, least costly, and safest thing that's available—which is you. There's no downside; the medical system is always there if you need it.

Considering the uncertain future of healthcare, it makes even more sense. No one knows what the healthcare system will look like in ten years, but few think we'll be getting better care at a lower price. The best way to use an uncertain healthcare system is the way we should have been using it all along—stay healthy and use it only when needed.

The cost of self-care is minimal. Except for the price of a few books, and an occasional seminar, it's free. Mostly, all it costs is your time. The risks are close to zero as well. You could fall off your chair as you're meditating, I suppose, but that's about as risky as it gets.

The only real risk relates to any medications you might be taking. As you eat better, exercise, and begin to meditate, your need for some types of medication will decrease. If you are currently on medication, you should check with your doctor before you begin any program of self-care. As you progress, you may need to have the dosage decreased—which should tell you something in itself.

Self-care also makes sense from a scientific point of view. Every cell in the body has thousands of receptors on the cell surface. They're like miniature docking stations waiting for a particular molecule to come along that fits. When one does, the two join like interlocking puzzle pieces. The interaction initiates a cascade of biochemical reactions within the cell. When the effect is multiplied by millions of similar cells, it results in physiologic change.

A pharmaceutical is a biochemical specifically designed to match a certain receptor. When introduced into the body, it binds with the receptor, causing the physiologic change that particular receptor is known to mediate—blood pressure goes up or down, urinary output increases or decreases, or bowel motility changes, depending on the drug.

Scientists are constantly racing to discover the next receptor so a drug can be quickly designed to match. There's a whole system involved. Patients get new treatment options, scientists' reputations are enhanced, and the bottom line of the pharmaceutical company gets a boost. Everybody wins.

A question they should be asking, however, is "What is the nature of the substance our body produces to interact with the receptor, and how can its production be enhanced?" There is no pharmaceutical that does not mimic a naturally occurring substance within the body. Every drug is a biochemical counterfeit.

This is the science upon which all self-care is based. There is little that a pill can do for us that we cannot also do for ourselves. A drug effect is stronger and more immediate than a natural effect, but it's also riskier. In the face of disease, pharmaceuticals can help right the ship. For disease prevention, it's safer if we learn to sail on our own.

Pharmaceuticals are miracles of modern technology, but they

are a mere shadow of the naturally occurring biochemical dance that exists within each one of us. Robert Blaich, M.D., coined the term "inner pharmacy" to describe this phenomenon and authored a book by the same name.

Most of our "inner drugs" flow automatically, but we have the ability to bring them under conscious control. With awareness and a little practice we can access our inner pharmacy whenever we want. It's a natural ability; we just have to remember how. This is the heart of self-care. And its power. It gives us more control over our health—and our lives—than we ever thought possible.

Me First: Is That Really Okay?

Somehow we've gotten the idea in our culture that putting ourselves first is selfish or self-indulgent. We've been told hundreds of times from a young age that "me first" simply isn't okay. But self-care isn't about hogging all the toys or making sure we're first in line for ice cream—the kind of "me first" our parents were talking about.

Self-care is about making sure our physical, emotional and spiritual needs are attended to, by the only person who can ever truly attend to them—us. Far from not caring about others, self-care is the firmest foundation from which we *can* authentically care for others.

As part of the flight attendant's safety briefing before every plane flight, we are instructed that if there's a mid-air emergency and the oxygen masks deploy, we should put our own mask on first before attending to any small children traveling with us. This may seem callous at first, but on closer inspection it makes perfect sense. If we put the child's mask on first, and we pass out from lack of oxygen, the child is left alone.

Is "me first" really okay? In terms of toys and ice cream, no. It's best to be polite and share. But in terms of our mental, physical, and spiritual health, it's not only okay, it's mandatory. Self-care is about understanding the importance of putting the oxygen mask on ourselves first. When we don't—everyone loses.

It's common for women, particularly mothers, to give to the point of exhaustion. Everyone always needs something, and they usually need it right now. Women are nurturing by nature and there is a strong tendency to take care of everyone but themselves. For short periods of time it's acceptable, and even beneficial to put others' needs before your own. Occasionally, life requires this. As a lifestyle, however, the effects can be damaging for you, and everyone around you.

What does this have to do with breast cancer? Possibly everything. The following personality traits are common to what W. Douglas Brodie, M.D. calls "the cancer-susceptible individual":[1]

1. Is highly conscientious, responsible, and hard-working.
2. Has a tendency to carry other people's burdens and take on extra obligations.
3. Has a deep-seated need to make others happy.
4. Harbors long-suppressed toxic emotions, especially anger and resentment.
5. Has an inability to resolve deep-seated emotional conflicts, often being unaware of their presence.
6. Is always willing to help, but reluctant to accept help from others.
7. Tends to "suffer in silence," bearing his or her burdens without complaint.

Many of us have some of these traits. But even if you have all of them it doesn't mean you're going to get cancer. What it means is that when our ideas about our responsibility to care for others are out of balance, it adversely affects our health—and we may not even be aware of it. For many of us, self-care begins when we stop trying to save the world.

The journey you are about to begin brings into focus the delicate balance between caring for yourself and caring for others. It will teach you how to put the oxygen mask on yourself first. It may seem strange at first because most of us aren't used to doing it. Developing the habit, however, will pay great dividends.

The importance of self-care is underscored by a pair of research studies done in the late 1970s by Harvard researchers Ellen Langer and Judith Rodin.[2,3] They divided nursing home residents into two different groups. Those in the first group were allowed to choose a plant and care for it any way they wished, to have a say in how the furniture in their room was arranged, and to choose which night they would see a movie. They were also given instructions on what to do if they had complaints.

Those in the second group were also given a plant but not allowed to choose which one. They were told the plant would be taken care of for them, and that the furniture in their rooms had already been arranged with their maximum comfort in mind. They were told which night they would see a movie, and given no mechanism to voice complaints.

After just a few weeks, those in the first group were judged to be happier, healthier, more social, and more alert. Astonishingly, a follow-up study eighteen months later found that of the residents who had since died, those in the "choice" group had lived an average of twice as long as those in the "no choice" group. Taking an active role in their own care not only enhanced their health, it also prolonged their life.

The parallels with breast cancer are unmistakable. The medical system encourages you to show up for your yearly mammogram and assures you that if you do, everything else will be taken care of. But while mammograms are helpful, and could save your life, it's better if you take more control than that. This book is meant to show you how.

Healing the Healer

If you are a physician, or working in the healthcare field in any capacity, don't forget that the self-care message applies to you too. As a healthcare professional who wants to help others, it's only natural to think of your patients as you learn about self-care techniques. That's great—they could all use it. But so could you.

If others are under your care in any capacity, they will benefit from a happier, healthier, more relaxed you. Put these techniques into effect in your own life before you "take them public." You can recommend them with greater authority if you speak from your own experience. In some ways you need them more than your patients.

Working in the healthcare system is highly stressful. U.S. physicians work longer hours than any other profession, have a higher divorce rate, and nearly double the suicide rate of the general population. One third of physicians would not go to medical school if they had it to do over again, and also advise their children not to go.[4] This is a staggering number considering the social and financial perks physicians enjoy in our society.

It begins early, with medical students routinely working 36-hour shifts, yet expected to be on top of their game at all times. The physical and emotional demands are extreme. It is an initiation like no other. There was a saying in medical school that "Medicine is the only animal that eats her own young." Anyone who's been though it knows exactly what that means.

After residency such long shifts are no longer required, but after years of training, the culture of overwork is set. It's bred into us. No one's driving us anymore, but we've learned to drive ourselves. Most of us have become quite good at it.

It isn't just physicians who suffer from the high-stress environment; all healthcare workers are affected. The stakes are high, the amount of scientific information is enormous, and perfection is required. Burnout—and sometimes worse—is common. If you are a healthcare worker, and you leave yourself out of the self-care equation, you have missed the point. If any of what follows makes sense to you, remember—you first. Then your patients. ◊

5
Eat Better, Feel Better, Live Longer

કે

A large part of putting the oxygen mask on ourselves first has to do with what we eat. Everything we put in our mouths either enhances our health or diminishes it. And it's a choice we all make at least three times a day. What you eat affects not only your breast cancer risk, but your risk of cancer in general. A major review of thousands of research studies on the relationship between diet and cancer concluded that roughly forty percent of *all* cancers could be prevented by proper nutrition.[1] Some think the number is even higher.

The question is, of course, "What *is* proper nutrition?" Hardly anyone seems to agree on the subject. There are thousands of diet books on the shelves telling us what to eat, but long before there were any books around, people were eating healthy. It can't possibly be as complicated as we make it.

The root of the problem is that the scientific community looks at food like they look at the human body—as the sum of its parts and nothing more. We have the technological means to identify some of the individual nutrients, and once we do, we set about analyzing each one to see which is "best."

This is referred to as reductionist philosophy, meaning that instead of considering the whole food an entity in itself, the focus is

43

on its individual nutrients. The thousands of individual substances that make up a whole food, such as an apple, are considered in isolation, as if they were not at all related to each other.

This is as limiting to our understanding of food as it is to our understanding of the human body. It's useful to look at things in detail as long as you keep the bigger picture in mind. But when you forget the bigger picture, the result is confusion—and often disaster.

From a reductionist point of view, there are two basic components of the diet: macronutrients and micronutrients. Macronutrients are those nutrients we need in relatively large amounts:

- carbohydrates
- fats
- proteins

Micronutrients are those nutrients we need in smaller amounts:

- vitamins
- minerals

Modern nutritional science and many diet books are primarily concerned with macronutrients. Up to a certain point this makes sense, since they are the building blocks of our food. But it's important to keep in mind that they're *only* building blocks. They're not the whole house. And they're not the whole neighborhood. They are an important part of the story—but not the entire story. A brief look at the macronutrients will reveal how confusing this approach can be.

Carbohydrates

The term "carbohydrate" refers to a food that contains carbon, hydrogen, and oxygen, a designation that is not very specific.

Eat Better, Feel Better, Live Longer

There's nothing in the term that differentiates a Snickers® bar from an apple, for instance, or a Twinkie® from a banana. These are all carbohydrates, even though there's a world of difference between them. The term carbohydrate, or "carb" as it is commonly known, is equivalent to "sugar," a term that's just as nebulous.

Since Snickers® bars, apples, Twinkies®, and bananas are all classified as carbs, many low-carb diets lump them all together. This is where common sense goes out the window in the name of science. Any first-grader, if given an apple, a banana, and a Twinkie®, could pick out the Twinkie® as being different. He may not be able to tell you *how* it's different, but he intuitively knows. As sensible adults, however, we rely more on our scientific institutions, often ignoring our deeper intuition. But as we've already seen, if we don't keep the paradigm of our scientific institutions in mind, we can easily be led down the garden path.

I was in our local organic market recently when someone introduced me to a woman with advanced breast cancer. She was walking up and down the produce aisle in an agitated state. "What am I supposed to eat!?" she wanted to know. "I can't have any of it! Everything has sugar in it." She had an array of the freshest local produce right in front of her, yet was full of anxiety because her doctor had told her sugar was bad for her. In giving her off-the-cuff nutritional advice, her doctor had lumped all sugars together, reflecting a deeper mindset that on a molecular level it's all the same: carbs are carbs. But this simply isn't so.

There's no question simple (processed) sugars are bad for you. Cancer is known to feed on these types of sugars. PET scans, the type of scan radiologists use for cancer staging, are based on sugar metabolism. The radioactive isotope used in PET scanning is biochemically attached to glucose in the laboratory, then injected into the patient. Once in the body, it goes wherever glucose goes. The radioactivity within the patient is then captured by detectors in the scanner and turned into an image. On the images, we're technically not seeing cancer. We're seeing sugar metabolism, which in a certain pattern is indicative of cancer. (figs 1,2)

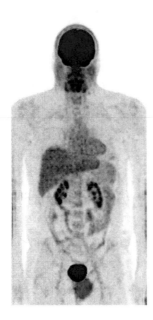

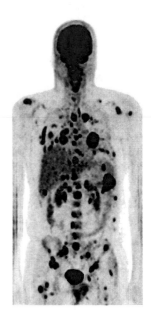

Fig. 1: Normal PET scan

Fig. 2: PET scan of the same patient three months later with widespread metastatic melanoma

Yes, we're using sugar to locate cancer, but it's pure glucose, injected intravenously. If we tagged the same radiopharmaceutical to an apple and had someone eat it, we couldn't diagnose anything even if they were riddled with cancer. Complex carbs from apples, pears, and so on, have fiber, vitamins, minerals, and thousands of other components. The body doesn't treat them the same as it does simple sugars.

Simple sugars depress the immune system and feed cancer. Complex sugars, as part of whole fruits and vegetables, enhance the immune system and fight cancer. Lumping fruits and vegetables in with processed sugar is worse than comparing the proverbial apples and oranges; it's comparing apples and Apple Cinnamon Pop Tarts®.

It doesn't even make medical sense to avoid all sugar, including fruits. Even if you never ingested another carb as long as you live, your blood sugar wouldn't go down to zero. You need sugar to live. If you quit eating carbs altogether, your body would just produce them on its own by cannibalizing healthy tissue.

Fats

The average American consumes roughly 40 percent of their daily calories from fat. The average Japanese diet contains just 9 percent fat. Scientists have long wondered if the low breast cancer rate in Japan might be due to their low-fat diet. Research studies seem to bear this out.

Women who have a diet low in fat get breast cancer less often than women who have a high-fat diet.[2] Of women with breast cancer, those who ate less fat prior to diagnosis had tumors that were smaller and had less evidence of tumor spread.[3] And women with low-fat diets live longer after diagnosis than women who have diets high in fat.[4]

Studies of women who reduce fat intake to 30 percent of total calories don't show this protective effect, but studies of women who reduce fat intake below 25 percent do.[5] And breast cancer is unheard of in populations that consume less than 10 percent of their daily calories as fat.[6]

The amount of fat consumed is not the only important factor to consider. The type of fat is important too. Unfortunately, this is where it gets complicated, because the term "fat" isn't any more specific than carbohydrate is. It doesn't differentiate between olive oil and lard, or between French fries and an avocado.

Fats are even more complicated than carbohydrates because of the greater variety of fats. There are saturated fats, unsaturated fats, polyunsaturated fats, and monounsaturated fats, as well as Omega-3 fats, Omega-6 fats, Omega-9 fats, and trans-fats. Some of these are healthy, some less healthy, and some extremely unhealthy.

At this point we will back away from following each macronutrient down its particular rabbit hole, and look at the bigger picture. Once we have a broader framework, all of this will make more sense. The key point to remember is that each macronutrient is only *part* of a food, not the whole food. Chasing each one individually, as if it weren't related to anything else, is missing the forest for the trees.

A Broader Perspective

As with most things in life, the problem with food lies in how we think about it. If we want to have a different relationship with food, we're going to have to think about it differently—more simply. At the most basic level, there are only two things to consider about food in terms of how it affects our health:

1. The nature of the food itself
2. What happens to it before it reaches our plate

Technically speaking, we don't eat carbohydrates, proteins and fats; we eat meat, fruits, vegetables, and grains. Even more basic than that, we eat either animal products or plants. Everything we consume is either an animal or a plant, or was derived from an animal or plant. The cancer picture as it relates to diet becomes clearer when we look at it in these simple terms.

What happens to our food before it reaches our plate can be further broken down into two categories: what happens to it on the farm, and what happens to it between the farm and us. The rest of our discussion then, will fall into the following categories:

1. Animal food vs. plant food
2. Whole food vs. processed food
3. Modern farming methods

We'll get back to our macronutrients, but we'll weave those discussions into this overall framework as we go along.

Animal Food vs. Plant Food

In a thirty-year study in rural China, described in his classic book, *The China Study,* Dr. T. Colin Campbell found that as the percentage of animal products in the diet rose, the breast cancer rate rose proportionately.[7] Laboratory research by Campbell and others has shown the same effect: rats fed a diet high in animal protein got breast cancer more often and died sooner than rats fed a lower percentage of animal protein. Rats fed a diet high in plant-based protein showed no increase in breast cancer.[8] This tells us that the body handles animal protein differently than plant protein—but it's not just about the protein.

Animals are made up of both fat *and* protein. You can't consume one without the other. Thus, it is impossible to know how much of the risk inherent in a high-fat diet is due to the meat, and how much of it is due to the fat—which is why we have to talk about food as a whole, not just its individual components.

Simply put, a healthy diet consists of large amounts of plants and fewer animals. Such a diet will reduce your risk of breast cancer, and other diseases as well. You may want to cut animal protein out altogether, but it's not necessary. Just reduce the amount. We don't need nearly the amount of protein the meat and dairy industry would like us to believe.

The U.S. government recommendation for daily consumption of protein is 0.8 grams per kilogram of body weight (1 kilogram is 2.2 lbs.), or about 10 to 15 percent of total daily calories. For a 110-pound woman, that's roughly 40 grams of protein per day. The World Health Organization recommendation is for half that: 0.45 grams per kilogram of body weight per day, or about 5 to 7 percent of total daily calories. According to the WHO, the same 110-pound woman would need just over 20 grams of protein per day.

Why the U.S. Government recommends twice the amount of protein in our daily diet as the WHO does is anybody's guess. Some think there are considerations involved other than just our health.

Whole Food vs. Processed Food

Whether from an animal or a plant, a "whole food" is food as it occurs in nature. Whole foods are the most nutritious foods. The only problem with them is that after a few days they go bad. Foods are "processed" so they will last longer on the shelf, making them more convenient. Processed foods are popular in modern culture because they're fast, easy—and cheap.

Almost anything that comes in a box or a wrapper falls into the category of a processed food. Processing involves removing part of the food and replacing it with preservatives, and/or artificial sweeteners. The problem is, it's usually the nutritious part that's removed.

Frank Oakes, owner Food and Thought, an organic grocery in Naples FL, says he knows of no change man has ever made to a food where the nutrition was actually enhanced. Every change has resulted in less nutrition, not more. In terms of processed foods, this can be true to the extreme.

Foods last longer on the shelf because bacteria won't eat them. But few of us stop long enough to wonder why. Bacteria don't eat processed foods because the nutritional value has been removed and replaced by foreign substances. In other words, eating these foods won't be good for them, and may even be harmful, so the bacteria don't waste their time on them.

Of all foods, perhaps the most highly processed is bread. Cakes, cookies, pastries, and many types of chips are all a form of bread product. A brief look at how bread is made is as enlightening as it is troubling.[9]

Bread is produced from flour, which is made from grains, most commonly wheat. A grain of wheat, sometimes known as a wheat berry, consists of three parts: the outer bran, the inner germ, and a starchy layer in between called the endosperm. The term "whole grain" refers to a grain that contains all three layers. Bread was traditionally made by milling or crushing the grain, making flour out of it, which is brown in color, and then baking bread from the flour. If you didn't use the flour within a few days, it went bad.

Refined flour is made only from the endosperm after separating out the bran and germ. This results in a fine, white flour that does not go bad. But the reason it doesn't go bad is that virtually all the nutrition is in the bran and the germ. Between thirty and forty nutrients and virtually all the fiber are removed by the refining process.

In addition, white flour is often bleached because this cuts the time between production and the grocery store shelf in half. The bleaching process, banned in many European countries, uses such chemicals as nitrogen oxide, chlorine, benzoyl peroxide, and potassium bromate, making the situation even worse for our health.

Refined, bleached flour and the products that come from them are some of the worst things we consume. From a nutritional standpoint it makes no sense. It only makes sense from a corporate profit standpoint. If these products were judged on their health benefits alone, they would be banned—and they almost were.

Shortly after white bread became widely available in the early 1900s, there was an increased incidence of pellagra and beriberi in the U.S. These are diseases of malnutrition, common in the third world, but exceedingly rare here. After investigation, the cause was attributed to the widespread availability of processed white bread.

Once its nutrient deficiencies were discovered, white bread no longer met the government standards for a food. To remedy the problem, manufacturers were required to put back five of the thirty to forty nutrients they had removed: niacin, thiamine, riboflavin, folic acid and iron. In adding back the five nutrients, food manufacturers were only doing what was required of them by law. Advertising these products as "enriched" or "fortified" is misleading at best.

Breakfast cereal is another example of a highly processed bread product. Breakfast cereals begin as whole grains, but by a high pressure, high temperature process known as extrusion, virtually all of the nutrition is destroyed.[10] Breakfast cereals are a multibillion-dollar business. They have been around for decades, but surprisingly, no studies have been done on their effects in humans. There are only two unpublished studies on rats.

In one of these studies, a group of rats was given water and a processed cereal to eat, while another group was given only water and the box. Astonishingly, *the rats that ate the box lived longer than the rats that ate the cereal*. In fact, the rats that ate the cereal died much sooner than expected.[11]

Breakfast cereals, like other highly processed foods, require extra enzymes, vitamins, and minerals from our bodies in order to be digested. There is a physiologic "cost" when we eat them because they contain virtually no enzymes, vitamins, or minerals of their own. Some of them are as much as fifty percent sugar. Literally, you're better off eating the box.

Food processing is an example of what happens when we try to improve on nature. In accomplishing exactly what we set out to do, we badly miss the mark. The food industry has achieved near immortality for their products, but the end result is like mummifying a human—it will last a long time, but there isn't any life in it.

Processed Food: The Consequences

The Western diet, high in such manipulated food products, is destructive to our health is three ways:

1. by the toxic effects of processed foods
2. by contributing to the obesity problem
3. by displacing healthier foods from our diet.

Refined sugar is highly concentrated, and is directly toxic to humans. A mere five ounces of refined sugar represents two and a half pounds of sugar beets.[12] The average American consumes 130 pounds of refined sugar yearly, which translates into nearly *half a ton* of sugar beets. Few humans could eat this many sugar beets in a lifetime, but thanks to the miracle of modern technology, we get the equivalent amount of sugar *every year.*

Consuming 100 grams (20 teaspoons) of processed sugar, roughly the amount in a 24 oz. soft drink, depresses immune function by fifty percent, with the effect lasting up to five hours.[13] This is a frightening fact considering that the average American consumes 20 teaspoons of added sugar *every day*, most of it hidden in cakes, cookies, soft drinks, and snack foods.[14]

This is important because the immune system is our primary

defense against cancer. Many experts believe we form cancer cells every day, but a healthy immune system recognizes these cells as foreign and disposes of them. From this point of view, the development of cancer occurs when a damaged or depressed immune system can no longer do its job. The fact that AIDS patients (known to have a debilitated immune system) routinely develop cancers that are rare in the general population would seem to substantiate this view.

Processed foods also contribute to the obesity problem. At the present time, fully two-thirds of the U.S. population is either overweight or obese.[15] Obesity rates have been rising rapidly for several decades and continue to rise regardless of age, gender, education level, or socio-economic status. The CDC refers to it as "the obesity epidemic." Obesity now poses as great a threat to our health as smoking, contributing to type 2 diabetes, heart disease—and cancer.[16]

Obesity is a known risk factor for breast cancer in post-menopausal women. The body's primary source of estrogen prior to menopause is the ovary, but after menopause it's fat. More fat stored in the body means higher levels of estrogen. Obese women who are post-menopausal have a sixty percent greater risk compared to women who maintain an ideal body weight.[17]

Of women diagnosed with breast cancer, obese women are twice as likely to die from it.[18] Scientists estimate that between 11,000 and 18,000 deaths per year in women over fifty could be avoided by maintaining an ideal body weight throughout adult life.[19] This is an astonishing statistic considering there are only 40,000 deaths from breast cancer each year.

And it isn't just about breast cancer. According to a 2003 article published in the New England Journal of Medicine, 14 percent of all cancer deaths in men, and 20 percent in women could be avoided by maintaining an ideal body weight.[20]

Processed foods contribute to obesity in many ways. Because of the very nature of these foods, it's difficult not to overeat. Processed foods are high in calories but low in nutrients and fiber. Whole foods, on the other hand, are high in nutrients and fiber, and low in calories. When you eat processed foods, these facts work against you. When you eat whole foods, they work in your favor.

A stomach full (approximately one liter) of potato chips, for example, contains roughly 3,000 calories. A stomach full of vegetables contains about 200 calories.[21] If you fill your stomach with either, it feels the same. Full is full, at least for a while. But because the potato chips are empty calories with virtually no nutrition or fiber, shortly afterward you're hungry again. On a mechanical level, you just ate, but on a cellular level you might as well not have because you provided your cells with little nutrition. So your body signals you to eat again, much sooner than if you had eaten something of nutritional value.

With a stomach full of vegetables you feel full longer because of the fiber content. Your body is also more satisfied because of the nutrition you just gave it, which theoretically is the reason we eat in the first place. You also consumed less than one-tenth the number of calories than if you had eaten the same volume of potato chips.

Health-wise, the vegetables are clearly the better deal. So why, when we sit down in front of the TV, do we so often grab for the chips and not the veggies? A big reason is right there on the TV screen. There are plenty of advertisements for chips, but virtually none for fruits and vegetables. Processed foods are about profitability, not your health.

Processed foods have largely displaced fruits and vegetables in the American diet—with disastrous results. The FDA recommends we get fifty to sixty percent of our daily calories from fruits, vegetables and whole grains. The average American gets only a fraction of that. For a 2,000 calorie-a-day diet, the Harvard School of Public Health recommends we get nine servings of fruits and vegetables per day.[22] Three-quarters of American families don't get five. Forty-five percent of people get *no* fruits in a day. Twenty-two percent get *no* vegetables in a day.[23] Even the few vegetables we *are* eating are dubious at best.

The three most commonly consumed vegetables in the U.S. are:

1. tomatoes in the form of catsup
2. potatoes in the form of French fries
3. iceberg lettuce

Why is the shift toward lower fruit and vegetable consumption so disastrous? Because of the nature of the fruits and vegetables. Nothing in the human diet has stronger cancer-fighting properties. Multiple studies show the incidence of all types of cancers to be lower in populations that eat large amounts of fruits and vegetables. Some experts even consider cancer a fruit and vegetable deficiency disease.[24] The following statement from a 1993 article published in Cancer Causes and Control sums it all up: "Vegetables and fruits contain the anti-carcinogenic cocktail to which we have become adapted. We abandon it at our peril."[25]

Not surprisingly, the substances in fruits and vegetables that help prevent cancer are the very things removed by food processing—most notably fiber, phytoestrogens, and antioxidants.

Fiber is the indigestible part of the plant. Technically it is not a nutrient, but it is a most important substance in terms of your health. Fiber gives food its bulk. In the stomach, this lets you know when it's time to stop eating. In the small bowel, it helps slow the absorption of sugars into the bloodstream. In the colon, it binds with estrogen and escorts it out of the body, decreasing estrogen levels.

Eat Better, Feel Better, Live Longer

Research studies exploring a possible link between a high-fiber diet and a decreased breast cancer risk have shown mixed results. Some studies show a large reduction in risk, while others show no effect at all. But regardless of breast cancer, a high-fiber diet is desirable for your general health. It is protective against colon cancer, diverticulitis, diabetes and heart disease. It lowers cholesterol as well as estrogen levels.

Fiber is not a food in itself; it is a marker of a healthy food. If a food is high in fiber it's good for you, period. Health experts recommend you get 35 grams of dietary fiber per day. The average American gets 10 to 15. In most non-industrialized countries the average intake is 50 to 70 grams per day. It is no coincidence that these countries have the lowest cancer rates.

Fruits and vegetables also contain *phytoestrogens*. These are plant-based estrogenic compounds, but are weaker than the estrogen your body produces. Phytoestrogens have a protective effect by binding to estrogen receptors and blocking the body's stronger estrogen from exerting its effects. Tamoxifen, the most well known of a class of drugs called SERMs (selective estrogen receptor modulators), decreases breast cancer risk by the same mechanism.

This is not to say you should throw out your Tamoxifen and replace it with an apple a day. But if you're taking Tamoxifen, why not eat in a way that may enhance its effects? And if you're not taking it, why not eat in a way that may offer some protection? A diet high in fruits and vegetables offers both.

Perhaps the most well known cancer-fighting substances in fruits and vegetables are *antioxidants*. Knowing what they are, and how they work, will help you understand how a diet high in fruits, vegetables, and whole grains can help prevent chronic disease.

Keep in mind that our discussion of fiber, phytoestrogens, and antioxidants is a detour back to the reductionist mindset. These substances provide us with a scientific basis for why fruits and vegetables have such powerful cancer-fighting properties, but none of them work in isolation. Separated from the food and ingested individually, they don't have the same effect.

Antioxidants, Free Radicals, and Oxidative Stress

In order to carry out life's basic processes, we must burn fuel for energy. Fuel is burned by a process called oxidation, and whether we're burning calories in our bodies, gasoline in our cars, or logs in the fireplace, the process is the same. The by-products of oxidation on the molecular level are called *free radicals*. Like smoke from a fire or the exhaust from your car, their production cannot be avoided. As long as we are alive and kicking we're burning fuel. And as long as we're burning fuel we are producing free radicals.

There are different kinds of free radicals, but one thing they all have in common is that they lack an electron. Like any positive ion in nature, free radicals seek to balance their electrical charge. A free radical, if not quickly neutralized, will attack our own bodies, in effect stealing an electron from healthy tissue, resulting in tissue damage.

Antioxidants are biochemical compounds that balance out the body's free radical production. Antioxidants provide the extra electron the free radicals crave. Our bodies manufacture a few antioxidants, but not nearly enough to stem the free radical tide. To do this, we must find them in our diet, which is where fruits and vegetables come in. Fruits and vegetables are the richest source of antioxidants in nature. When we consume them in adequate amounts, their antioxidants neutralize free radicals before they can accumulate in the body and cause damage.

The formula is simple: An adequate amount of fruits and

vegetables in our diet provide plenty of antioxidants to neutralize free radical production, leaving our bodies healthy. A low intake of fruits and vegetables allows free radicals to predominate, damaging our cellular structure in unpredictable ways, a situation called *oxidative stress*.

Oxidative stress explains why so many seemingly unrelated diseases can result from a poor diet. The disease process depends upon which healthy tissue is damaged by the free radicals. DNA damage causes mutations that can result in cancer. Damage to the nerve sheath can result in multiple sclerosis. Damage to the inner lining of blood vessels causes plaque formation that can result in a heart attack or stroke. Inflammation is well known to be an underlying cause of many different diseases. Oxidative stress causes the inflammation.

The fireplaces in our homes are beneficial. They provide light and keep us warm. But when the chimney is stopped up, smoke fills the house and the same fire which *was* a benefit, now becomes deadly. Not eating enough fruits and vegetables is like stopping up the chimney.

It's also like stopping up the exhaust pipe in your car. People commit suicide this way because the carbon monoxide in the exhaust displaces oxygen in the blood. While breathing deeply, they suffocate to death. Free radicals won't suffocate us like carbon monoxide will, but the mechanism is similar in terms of a harmful chemical reaction involving a waste product that wasn't properly disposed of. Over time, the outcome is the same: A chronically poor diet, continued for years, is slow suicide.

We don't see the effects immediately because each free radical hit on a healthy cell is a sub-microscopic event, one among multiple trillions taking place all the time. Each hit is like throwing a stone at a 747 sitting on a runway. Nothing much appears to be happening on a gross level. But continue throwing stones at it 24/7 for thirty, forty, or fifty years, and it will eventually break down—as do our bodies when we live in a state of chronic oxidative stress.

Our culture tells us that at fifty, sixty, or seventy years of age, our bodies naturally begin to break down and we get the expected diseases of aging: arthritis, diabetes, heart disease, and cancer. But nothing could be further from the truth. A study of any indigenous society will tell you these are *not* the usual diseases of aging. They can't be, or everyone in the world would get them at more or less the same age, which they don't. These are lifestyle diseases, rare in the third world, in large part because the third world eats differently than we do.

It is a little known but sobering fact, that the mechanism of tissue injury from a poor diet is the same as that caused by radiation—free radical damage.[26] Whether a free radical is produced by a normal biochemical process, or by an electron knocked out of its orbital shell by a photon of X-ray energy is immaterial to the free radical. Regardless of how it was "born," it sets about its business of eating up electrons from neighboring healthy tissue—unless there are enough antioxidants around to feed its cravings.

This is not meant to raise anxiety. You don't get cancer from occasional exposure to low-dose medical radiation, and you don't get it from eating a few doughnuts once in a while. The effects of both are like throwing stones at the 747. The point is, we have a healthy respect for radiation, but we're much more cavalier about the food. We shouldn't be.

Supplements

This is a good time to discuss nutritional supplements, not only because they contain antioxidants, but also because supplements mirror our processed food discussion. There is as much confusion about supplements as there is about the food. And for the same reasons. The terms "vitamin" and "antioxidant" are no more specific than the terms carbohydrate and fat. Labeling a substance as one or the other doesn't tell you what it is.

An apple, for instance, contains thousands of different biochemical compounds (phytochemicals), one of which we have identified and labeled Vitamin C, an antioxidant.[27] The Vitamin C tablet you find in the drug store is also an antioxidant, but the two are not at all the same.

One serving of apple (100 grams) contains about 6 mg. of Vitamin C, but tests show that the antioxidant power of the apple is equivalent to *1,500* mg of Vitamin C in tablet form.[28] It would seem that the Vitamin C in the apple is more potent than that of the tablet, but the Vitamin C component of the apple accounts for less than one percent of the apple's total antioxidant capacity.

What contributes the rest of it? Nobody knows. The Vitamin C in the apple is in its natural state as part of the whole food. It works as part of the synergy of the whole in a way that's too complex for us to understand. The majority of the phytochemicals in the apple are yet to be identified. We don't even know what they are, much less what they do, or how they interrelate. It's *so* complex it becomes simple—the apple is always a better choice than the drug store tablet.

There are two basic types of nutritional supplements. The first is based on whole food. Though we often refer to them as such, these are not technically supplements; they are whole food concentrates. Whole food concentrates usually consist of some combination of fruits and vegetables dehydrated to a powder form. They aren't the whole food, but they're a reasonable facsimile. The magic of the whole food, which lies in the synergy of all its parts, is largely preserved.

Chapter Five

The other type of supplement is referred to as a "fragmented" vitamin. The drug store Vitamin C tablet is an example. It's called fragmented because it doesn't contain all the other ingredients that occur with vitamin C in nature. It's only a fragment of the whole food. Multivitamins are another type of fragmented vitamin. There may be up to 100 different vitamins and minerals in a multivitamin tablet, but that's only a fraction of what's in the food. And the 100 you're getting are not in the same proportion as they occur in nature. Fragmented vitamins are the nutritional supplement equivalent of a highly processed food—the majority of the "good stuff" has been removed.

The following, adapted from Dr. Mitra Ray's *From Here to Longevity*, is a good illustration of the difference between whole food or whole food concentrates, and fragmented vitamins:[29]

What your body sees with the vitamin:

```
    T ke    r ght  n Gr  n St   t. G  t  th  f rst
tr ff   l ght  nd st y  n th  l ft l n  t  m k
a    ft  n M ntg m ry Bl d. P ss thr    st p s gns
 nd f ll w c rv d r  d  p th  h ll t  th  f  rth
st p s gn. M k  r ght  n M ch g n Str   t.
```

What your body sees with whole food:

```
    Take a right on Green Street. Go to the first
traffic light and stay in the left lane to make
a left on Montgomery Blvd. Pass three stop signs
and follow curved road up the hill to the fourth
stop sign. Make a right on Michigan Street.
```

Apples and the human body are perfectly adapted to each other. A fragmented vitamin is incomplete, often synthetic, and concentrated to levels the human body was never meant to see. The body intuitively knows what to do with the food. With the fragmented vitamin, it's not so sure.

There is no government recommendation either for or against taking nutritional supplements for disease prevention. This is because the research on the subject is inconclusive. Considering that few studies specify what kinds of supplements are being taken, this comes as no surprise. In most studies, supplement usage is specified only as the patients taking "multivitamins" or "antioxidants," which could mean almost anything.

Researchers tend to treat supplements as if the exact makeup doesn't matter. But it *does* matter. The difference between a whole food concentrate and a fragmented vitamin can be as large as the difference between a potato and a potato chip, or a grape and a purple jellybean. It is an exact parallel of our whole food vs. processed food discussion. In the whole food concentrate, the magic of the food remains largely intact. In the fragmented vitamin, the synergy is lost.

Most studies on multivitamin usage show no positive effect, and some even show a harmful effect. A recent study from Sweden showed a twenty percent increase in breast cancer risk in women who took multivitamins.[30] This is a "relative risk", something we will discuss in a later chapter, so the danger is not as great as it might seem. But the question remains, if these products are mostly not helpful and may be harmful, why take them?

Research studies on whole food concentrates tell a different story. Studies on one whole food concentrate* show a significant decrease in DNA fragmentation and enhanced immunity in people taking it for even a short period of time.[31,32] This is highly significant

* Juice Plus+®

63

because DNA integrity and the strength of our immune system are two important pillars of cancer prevention.

If you choose to take some type of supplementation, broad-spectrum fruit and vegetable concentrates are the best choice for general health and disease prevention. They're not the whole food, but they're the next best thing. They are the most logical, effective, and safest way to make up for what is lacking in our modern food supply.

The Modern Farm

Our food supply has changed more in the last fifty years than it has in the last ten thousand.[33] Farming methods have changed so drastically in the last few decades it has given rise to the term "factory farm." The food we eat in the industrialized world is, not surprisingly, increasingly industrialized.

Very little of our food comes from the idyllic family farm of our grandparents' days. The factory farm has largely pushed the family farm out of existence. The factory farm has literally changed the way America eats—yet most of America isn't aware of it.

The biggest differences between today's farm and its counterpart of half a century ago involve the use of chemical pesticides, artificial fertilizers, and modern methods of meat and dairy production. These result in higher yields and cheaper food, but come at a price of less nutrition and higher exposure to toxic chemicals.

Over a billion pounds of *chemical pesticides* were used in the U.S. in 2001, the last year for which statistics are available.[34] This represents 25 percent of the world's yearly production. In terms of their effect on our health, pesticides are classified as either "xenoestrogens" or "endocrine disruptors." Xenoestrogens are foreign substances that act like estrogen when introduced in the human body.

The term "endocrine disruptor" is fairly self-explanatory. Both upset the delicate balance of your hormonal system, which in turn affects your breast cancer risk.

Large scale *artificial fertilizer* use began shortly after World War II, when there were huge stockpiles of nitrogen-based explosives left over from the war. In order not to waste them someone came up with the idea of using them as fertilizer. Cow manure, which is traditionally used as fertilizer, is also high in nitrogen, so it seemed logical. The problem is, the soil reacts differently to artificial fertilizer than it does cow manure.

Artificial fertilizers result in high yields initially, but because they kill the microflora in the topsoil, they destroy the soil's ability to sustain itself. This requires ever-increasing amounts of fertilizer to maintain the same crop yield, which results in a slow degradation of the nutrient value of the soil—which results in a slow degradation of the nutrient value of anything *grown* in the soil. Soil erosion and mineral depletion result in $20 billion worth of plant nutrients lost from agricultural soils every year.[35]

The third major area where modern farming methods affect us, and possibly the worst in terms of breast cancer risk, involves the *meat and dairy industry.* The overwhelming majority of beef cattle in the U.S. are fed corn. Because of government subsidies on corn, it's cheaper to feed cattle corn than it is grass, even though grass is what cows normally eat.

Ninety-five percent of corn in the U.S. is genetically modified (GM) to be resistant to pesticides. This results in much higher pesticide use than was previously the case, since higher concentrations can be used without fear of killing the corn. Commercial pesticide use has increased 33 fold in the last two decades, which parallels the virtual takeover of GM corn.[36]

Pesticides are lipophilic, meaning they are preferentially stored in fat. They are stored in the fat of the cows after they eat the corn, and then stored in your fat after you eat the cows—effectively raising your estrogen levels. In addition, milk cows are given hormones to increase production, and beef cattle are given steroids to increase bulk. Both are passed along to you when you eat the meat or drink the milk, raising your estrogen levels even more.

To most of us, the food chain has only two links: the grocery store and us. But just because we're not aware of the rest of the food chain doesn't mean we're not affected by it. We tend to forget that for animal food, we're eating the animal *and* whatever it ate.

It is a well-known biologic phenomenon that toxic substances become more concentrated as they go up the food chain. Thus, pesticides become more toxic to us when they are concentrated in animal fat than they would be if we ate them directly from the plants. If we eat a few ears of corn, we are exposed only to the pesticides on the corn we've eaten. Beef cattle, on the other hand, eat tons of corn in their short lifetimes, and concentrate the pesticides from all of it in their fat. And when you eat the cow, it gets concentrated in yours.

Women who have breast cancer have a higher level of these chemicals in their breast tissue than women who do not.[37] More studies need to be done, but chemical estrogens appear to be far more dangerous than the general public suspects.

Collateral Damage

Estrogenic pesticides don't just affect the food; they affect the water as well. And the effect is not limited to the farm. Because of the runoff from pesticides and fertilizers washing down the Mississippi River from Midwestern farmland, there is a "dead zone" in the Gulf of Mexico just off the Louisiana coast for several months each year where no life exists.[38] It is essentially "collateral damage" from modern farming practices.

The size of the dead zone varies from year to year, but it often involves over a hundred square miles. A common sense question brings the chemical pesticide and artificial fertilizer issue into perspective: Are we really to believe that substances which kill every living thing hundreds of miles distant from where they were used—despite being diluted by trillions of gallons of water—don't also adversely affect us?

The modern farm is a major vehicle for toxic chemicals to reach us, but it's not the only vehicle. It was recently discovered that the drinking water at Camp Lejeune, a Marine base in North Carolina, was highly contaminated with industrial chemicals for over twenty years.[39] To date, 70 men who were stationed there during that time have since been diagnosed with breast cancer. This is an unheard of number of male breast cancer cases.

The Camp Lejeune male breast cancer cluster is the largest ever reported. Studies are underway to determine if the contaminated water was truly the cause, but don't wait for the outcome of the study; find a source of pure drinking water now. It will protect you from this type of environmental disaster. Filtered water alone won't do it. Charcoal filters take care of large contaminants, but estrogens in the water are too small to be filtered out.

Many consider toxic chemicals in the environment to be a time bomb waiting to go off. These chemicals are ubiquitous, occurring in plastics, cleaning products, make-up, and hair products, to name just a few. Many of these chemicals are strongly suspected to have a causative effect on breast cancer.

The Breast Cancer Fund, a non-profit organization based in San Francisco, is a leading voice in raising awareness of environmental causes of breast cancer. Their website has a wealth of information on the subject. (www.thebreastcancerfund.org)

Chapter Five

Macronutrients Revisited

Now that we have a better framework for how to look at food, it's time to revisit our macronutrients to see how they fit. The confusing carbohydrate picture becomes exceedingly clear when we look at it from a whole food vs. processed food perspective. It isn't about the carbs; it's about the integrity of the food. A whole food is an entity unto itself, and cannot be manipulated without unintended consequences.

The complex subject of fats also becomes simple when approached from the standpoint of animal vs. plant food, whole vs. processed food, and modern farming methods. You can study the table on the following page at your leisure, but what it tells us is exactly what we would expect: animal fats increase breast cancer risk, while plant fats decrease it; chemically processed oils increase risk, while mechanically processed oils (olive oil) decrease it; and the most dangerous oils (trans-fats) are the ones that have been the most chemically manipulated. It even speaks to modern farming methods: wild (not farm-raised) salmon contain healthy fats, as does grass-fed (not corn-fed) beef.

Eat Better, Feel Better, Live Longer

Fats and Breast Cancer Risk

TYPE OF FAT	SOURCE	EFFECT ON RISK	MECHANISM OF RISK
Saturated Fats:			
Saturated fats:	Animal products	⬆ Risk	⬆ Estrogen levels
Unsaturated Fats: (mostly from *plant sources*)			
Monounsaturated fats:			
Omega-9 Fats:	Olive oil*	*Protective effect*	*Enhance immunity*
Polyunsaturated fats:			
Omega-3 fats:	(whole foods) Flaxseeds Walnuts Avocados Deep water fish (salmon, halibut) Grass-fed beef	*Protective effect*	*Enhance immunity Anti-inflammatory*
Omega- 6 fats:**	(highly processed) Corn oil Sunflower oil Safflower oil Soy oil	⬆ Risk	Degrade immunity Inflammatory
Trans fats:***	(artificial) Fried foods Chips Cookies Margarine	⬆⬆ Risk	Unknown

* Mechanically, not chemically processed

** These fats are healthy as part of the natural plants. They're unhealthy in the highly processed oils

*** The most dangerous fats; significantly increase breast cancer risk
Produced by chemical manipulation of already highly processed Omega-6 oils
Also known as "partially hydrogenated oils"
Banned in some European countries, and some states in the U.S.

Chapter Five

Do I Really Need to Eat Organic?

Yes, if at all possible. It will protect you from the majority of the ills of factory farming. Eating organic is considered to be a fad by some, but all of our grandparents ate organic because that's all there was. It is a sign of the times that we've come up with a new term to describe eating how *everyone* used to eat.

One of the complaints about organic food is the cost. It may seem like semantics, but organic food isn't more expensive; conventionally grown food is artificially cheaper. Sure, you can get a higher yield if you blanket the soil with artificial fertilizer, spray the crops with chemical pesticides, feed the cows government-subsidized corn, and inject them full of hormones so they'll grow bigger, faster. A higher yield means a cheaper product. But is it really cheaper?

If you consider the cost per calorie, organic food does cost more. But if you consider the cost per *nutrient*, the cost of conventionally grown food is astronomically higher. Like everything you buy, the main consideration isn't price—it's value. If you're paying more, what are you getting for the extra cost? Organic food is a better value than conventional food, both in terms of what you get (more nutrients), and what you don't get (the estrogenic effects of pesticides, hormones, etc.). Organic food costs more because it's more labor intensive, and it's grown with more care. It's worth it.

To Sum Up

We've covered a lot of ground in this chapter, but it needn't be overwhelming. The majority of the information presented has been either to raise awareness about the state of our food supply, or to provide a scientific basis for diet and cancer prevention. As far as what you should eat, it's simple.

Eat Better, Feel Better, Live Longer

Just a few dietary changes will protect you from virtually all of the risk inherent in today's food supply. If you do the following, you can practically forget all the details. You don't have to be an organic chemist or a food detective to eat healthy. You just have to think about food differently.

- Eat real (not processed) food.

- Eat mostly plants. About 90 percent plant food and 10 percent animal products is the ideal mix, but nothing is set in stone. It's what you do most of the time that matters most.[40]

- Eat organic if at all possible, and if you can't, at least eat grass-fed beef. Pay more for it and eat less of it. This will enhance your health and be budget neutral.

- Drink lots of pure water. This will help maintain an ideal body weight, reduce collateral damage from the factory farm, and protect you from other hidden environmental dangers as well.

- Eat healthy as much as possible, and don't stress out about it when you don't. Stress is counterproductive to everything you're trying to accomplish. As we will see in the following chapter, stressing out about your health is a very *un*healthy thing to do. ❧

6

What About All the Stress?

❧

The altering of the food supply and the increase in the number of toxic chemicals in the environment in the last fifty years is unprecedented. Many feel the dramatic rise in cancer incidence during the same period is no coincidence. But the physical part of our environment—the food we eat, the water we drink, the air we breathe—is only part of the picture. The world is becoming an increasingly complex place to live on many levels.

The amount of information available to us that wasn't available to our grandparents is staggering. A weekday edition of the New York Times contains more information than the average person was likely to come across in a lifetime in seventeenth century England.[1] The amount of knowledge in the biological sciences doubles every six months, and the amount of electronic information available doubles faster than that.[2] Information is now so abundant it is a matter of concern. According to John L. King, Dean of the University of Michigan School of Information, "We're drowning in it."

We have to assimilate all this information just like we have to digest our food. In a sense, we have to mentally digest everything that happens to us. And a lot of it is harmful. Just as there are unhealthy foods, there are unhealthy thoughts and perceptions. Just as there are toxic chemicals, there are toxic emotions. What we see, think, and feel affects us on a deeper level than most realize.

In a Western medical paradigm that considers the body simply the sum of its mechanical parts, it's understandable how something as mysterious as the human mind can be so confounding. Despite our modern technology, no one knows what the mind actually is. But whatever the mind is, it's clear that it affects every aspect of our biology. And nowhere is the mind's power to affect the body more evident than in the area we call stress.

The rate of stress-induced illness has skyrocketed in recent years. Cardiologist Robert Eliot, M.D., author of *Is It Worth Dying For?* calls stress "the largest contributor to illness in the industrialized world." More than 75% of all doctor's visits in the United States are due to stress-related illnesses.[3] Many in Western medicine do not acknowledge a mind-body connection, but the stress-related illness statistics make clear that there is one.

The possible link between stress and breast cancer is something we have already touched on. Some studies show an increased incidence of breast cancer in women who describe themselves as chronically stressed, and women who have experienced recent traumatic life events may also be at increased risk.[4,5]

Not all studies show a link between stress and breast cancer incidence, but the damaging effects of stress are bigger than breast cancer. You don't win the game if you manage to avoid breast cancer, but die an early death from a heart attack or stroke. Minimizing your stress *may* decrease your risk of breast cancer, but it is certain to decrease your risk of everything else. Learning to deal effectively with stress is one of the most beneficial things you can do for your health.

What About All the Stress?

The Stress Response

Most of us have an intuitive understanding of what stress is, but it can be surprisingly difficult to define. The term "stress" was originally a physics term referring to an outside force applied to a body. It is a measure of how much force a material can withstand before it breaks down.

Harvard professor William Bradford Cannon first described biological stress in the 1920s calling it "the fight-or-flight response." He noted that this occurred in all vertebrates when an external threat was perceived. He also found that no matter what the threat was, the physiologic response was the same.

The response is one of arousal and preparation for action: Heart rate and breathing accelerate, blood pressure is elevated, the pupils dilate, and blood is shunted away from the brain and digestive tract and redirected to the large muscles.

This all makes perfect sense if we think of a primitive human walking through the jungle and suddenly seeing a bear. He doesn't need to think or digest; he needs to run or fight. He needs more oxygen fast to do either one, and he needs to see clearly in case other predators are nearby. His body's stress response prepares him for action.

When the threat no longer exists, the stress response reverses, bringing the body back into what we call homeostasis. Breathing, heart rate and blood pressure normalize, blood is shunted back into the brain and digestive organs, and the pupils return to normal.

Both of these responses—the arousal and the return to equilibrium—are mediated by the autonomic nervous system (ANS), whose job it is to maintain a stable internal environment. The ANS has two distinct parts: the sympathetic nervous system, and the parasympathetic nervous system. The sympathetic nervous system prepares us for action through "the fight-or-flight response." The parasympathetic system returns us to equilibrium through what has been called "the relaxation response."

The two systems are complementary. They work together, allowing us to respond to a threat when the need arises, but maintain a stable internal environment otherwise. The sympathetic system can be thought of as the gas pedal on your car; it engages when you need to go—now. The parasympathetic system can be thought of as the brakes; it engages when you need to slow down. This complex physiologic dance occurs automatically, without you having to think about it, hence the name "autonomic."

Our primitive human scenario describes a situation we call *acute stress*. A threat occurs, an appropriate response is made, and things quickly return to normal. In modern life, this would be equivalent to a sporting event. When runners are on the blocks ready for a big race to begin, the same physiologic events occur that we've just described. Pulse and blood pressure rise, blood is shunted to the large muscles, and so on.

When the starter's pistol goes off, they race down the track, and shortly after crossing the finish line, their bodies return to a normal state. A bear could have been chasing them; their bodies don't know the difference. But bear or no bear, acute stress is actually good for us. There are a number of health benefits, not the least of which is a strengthening of the immune system.

Building on Walter Cannon's work, Wilhelm Raab discovered the hormones cortisol and adrenaline which, when released by the adrenal glands in response to sympathetic discharge, cause the physiologic changes of the fight-or-flight response. He also discovered that these hormones, which are beneficial in intermittent doses, become toxic when the body is exposed to them for long periods.

It is the long-term situation we call *chronic* stress that is so bad for our health. Hans Selye, another Harvard researcher, later showed that chronic stress can cause disease in both animals and humans. It was Selye who popularized the word stress. Cortisol and adrenaline became known as "stress hormones."

There aren't many bears around today, but there are plenty of uncooperative spouses, overbearing bosses, and an ever-increasing supply of anxiety-provoking events on the news. Many of us ruminate on these things, holding them in our minds long after the event is over. We worry about imagined threats that don't actually exist in the moment. Physiologically, this is the equivalent of the bear being present all the time.

The Nature of Stress

Now that we understand how stress affects our bodies, it's time to get back to a definition. Claire Wheeler, M.D., Ph.D., author of *10 Simple Solutions to Stress,* describes stress as a process—an interaction between a person and the environment. Stress is the situation that occurs when life's challenges and pressures outstrip a person's ability to cope with them. In other words, stress is a balance between what happens and how you respond to it.

This explains why getting a scientific handle on stress can be so difficult. What's stressful for you may not be stressful for me, and vice versa. Not only that, what I find stressful today may not be stressful for me tomorrow because my ability to cope might be better then.

Understanding that fully half the definition of stress has to do with us is a giant step toward better stress management. Mental and emotional stresses, the most common types in our society, have no meaning outside the human mind. The environment exists. Stuff happens, as they say. But without someone to interact with the stuff—to interpret it if you will—there can be no stress. In biological terms, stress can only exist within the interpreter.

The significance of events will vary from person to person, but in general, events such as having our car stolen will carry more significance than spilling our soup. On a practical level, when the significance of daily events is equal to our ability to cope with them, we're having a pretty good day. When the events of the day are beyond our ability to cope, our day is more challenging. And when our ability to cope exceeds whatever happens, it's a great day. This can be expressed algebraically as follows:

A Good Day: Significance of events = our ability to cope
A Bad Day: Significance of events > our ability to cope
A Great Day: Significance of events < our ability to cope

Breaking things down further, we see that the significance of an event itself is a two-fold process, half of which again has to do with us. There's the actual event, and our perception of the event, which is the meaning or significance we give to it. This puts even more of the stress equation within our reach.

Significance of event = the event + our perception of it.

If a good friend walks by me at the mall and says nothing, my thinking can follow several paths: "I wonder if Mary's mad at me. Maybe I've upset her in some way." Or "I know Jim had a doctor's appointment this morning. Maybe he got bad news." Or "That was rude! I know he saw me. Bill said he was a friend, but now I'm beginning to wonder."

The only thing I really know is that Mary, Jim, or Bill walked by without saying anything. That is a fact. Everything else is my interpretation, a story I tell myself about the event—*which may or may not be true.* Depending on what my story is, I might experience stress over the event or I might not.

I might begin to analyze every word I've said to Mary over the last week that could have caused her to be upset with me. I might be so concerned about Jim that I call to see if everything is okay. Or I might feel so insulted by Bill's snub that I won't talk to him for a month. It's the path my mind takes that determines how much stress I feel, not the event itself.

Stress then, is always based on three factors:

1. An event
2. The meaning I give to the event
3. My coping skills

As long as I keep these factors in mind, I have a good chance of dealing effectively with the stresses in my life. The problem comes when I forget about the last two and consider events stressful in and of themselves. Unfortunately, this is how most of the culture defines stress.

We talk about stressful people, stressful situations at work, and stressful events, but rarely do we consider our part in the equation. In our mall scenario, I might describe to a friend how Bill or Mary stressed me out this morning. Jim, however, is still a great guy—at least in my mind—even though he did exactly the same thing as the others.

Some events, like the attacks on the World Trade Center, seem so much larger than life that we consider them stressful in and of themselves. But while most in our part of the world were grieving, some in other parts of the world were dancing in the streets. Why? Because the meanings attached to the event were wildly different.

The Talmud says, "We do not see the world as it is, we see the world as we are," which is a perfect description of the paradigm effect. Our paradigms, perspectives, and points of view are so deeply ingrained we rarely question them—but we should. Our paradigms are the lens through which we view even the most powerful events. But the lens can be adjusted. In the stress equation, events are the constant. *We* are the variable.

Events are facts. In the strictest sense, they are always neutral. Everything in my mind that follows an event is an opinion. It is only my unquestioning belief in my opinions that makes them seem so solid. But what seems solid to me may not have any basis in reality. And when it doesn't, I will experience stress.

Our mall scenario makes it clear that much of our stress is self-inflicted. If I never consider that my own perspective is part of what's causing my stress, I will never grow beyond my present ability to manage stress. This gives away much of my personal power, and assures I will stay stuck in whatever perspective I have at the moment, whether it benefits me or not. It puts events in control of me instead of the other way around.

Appropriate vs. Inappropriate Control

We generally don't experience stress unless we feel a loss of control. And there is no better way to feel out of control than to consider people, events, and situations inherently stressful without giving any consideration to our part in the process.

This gives away the only part of the game we have control over—ourselves—and focuses on the part we don't—outside events and other people. It's natural for us to try to regain control if we think we've lost it, but there are two distinctly different paths we can take in our attempts to do so. One alleviates stress. The other only causes more.

What About All the Stress?

If, after determining I cannot change a situation, I focus on my attitude and finding more effective ways to cope with it, my stress will begin to subside. It may not go away immediately, but at least I'm heading in the right direction. If, however, I have no awareness of my part in the process, I will try to control the people and situations around me in order to diminish my stress. Since I have no power to control those things, this only adds to the stress I already feel.

A good metaphor for the issue of appropriate vs. inappropriate control is the proverbial "getting our ducks in a row." This is a phrase commonly used to describe our efforts to put things in their proper order, which usually means requiring those around us to line up with *our* idea of what proper order is. In terms of stress, this is an accident waiting to happen—for everyone concerned. I may be the driver, but it will be more than a single car crash.

When we look closer, the picture of the mother duck crossing the road with her baby ducklings following behind in a neat little row tells us something entirely different. The mother duck never scurries about in a frenzy—pushing, cajoling, or otherwise coercing the ducklings to stay in line. In fact, she never looks back at all. Presumably, she has already taken care of things in terms of feeding and nurturing, so when it's time to cross the road, all she has to do is lead the way and the ducklings naturally follow.

In other words, having taken care of what is within her power to control, she lets everything else take care of itself. The mother duck's demeanor as she crosses the road is one of calm assurance. She is not stressed, even though her ducklings are at great risk if they run off.

This is the major skill necessary in dealing with *any* kind of stress, but is particularly useful in the breast cancer issue. Whether you're looking for prevention, end up having to deal with terminal cancer, or anything in between, the skill necessary is the same: *Focus on the things you have control over and don't waste any time or energy on what you don't.*

Stating the same thing another way:

> God grant me the serenity
> to accept the things I cannot change;
> courage to change the things I can;
> and wisdom to know the difference...

There's a reason this is called the *Serenity Prayer.* Understanding the difference between what we can change and what we cannot is the only way we can have serenity. And serenity is the only place from which we can recognize the difference.

When we stray outside of ourselves, trying to control things we have no power to control, we will feel stress. When we stay within ourselves, looking to the only things we *can* control—our own perceptions and attitudes—we can remain at peace, even in the most difficult of circumstances.

Stress and Breast Cancer

Unlike the chronic stresses of everyday life, much of the stress surrounding breast cancer is acute in nature. It's uncomfortable, but it won't kill you. It may be terrifying, but it's temporary. A screening mammogram is a once-a-year event; an abnormal mammogram result is much less common; and the need for a biopsy is rarer still.

Short of a cancer diagnosis, these events appear for a time and then recede into the background. Managing the stress that surrounds them will be helpful, but not life saving, because this is not the kind of stress that kills you. Even the stress of a cancer diagnosis, terrifying as it may be, is a type of acute stress.

What About All the Stress?

For the survivor, it is a different story. A survivor must endure an underlying, low-level stress that few others understand. When every headache and muscle cramp might be a sign the cancer has returned, it presents a special challenge.

High-risk women face a similar challenge. When every woman in your family has been diagnosed with breast cancer, it's hard not to feel like it's only a matter of time for you. This type of chronic stress can be difficult to deal with, and is debilitating for some. It affects women deeply, often below their level of awareness.

Dealing with the unique mix of stresses surrounding breast cancer may seem like a daunting task, but once you understand the nature of stress, it becomes quite simple. It's not necessarily *easy*. But it's simple. You confront any stress by working with the only parts of the stress equation within your control: your perceptions and your coping skills.

Having an abnormal mammogram or needing a biopsy are just facts. Being at high risk or being diagnosed are facts. The fears lying one step deeper are the crux of the matter: "Am I going to need a mastectomy?" "Is my husband going to still find me desirable?" "Am I going to die?" "What's going to happen to the kids?" Or for high-risk women, "When is the hammer going to fall?"

On the surface, these seem like issues unique to women, but they're not. Breast cancer—or the specter of it—forces a woman to deal with things all of us should be dealing with: our self-image, the quality of our relationships, our mortality, and the uncertainties of life. These can be uncomfortable issues to confront, but once you do, a certain peace begins to emerge. It doesn't show up all at once; it comes as you are willing to confront the issues.

While you are waiting for more peace to show up, there is still much you can do to diminish your stress, namely work on your coping skills. Again, this isn't necessarily easy, but it's simple.

Chapter Six

Remember, there are many kinds of stress, but only one physiologic response. Master that physiologic response, and you master life—breast cancer or not.

You can master the physiologic stress response by developing "mind-body skills," so named because they are mental skills that positively affect your physical health. Because modern stress is largely a mental phenomenon, they attack it at its source.

The rest of the book will touch on the deeper issues of life, as well as help you build a practical toolkit of mind-body skills. The information presented will help you be less emotionally reactive to events outside of your control, and show you what *is* within your control. It will help you deal with any stress, including that surrounding the mammographic process. It will help you navigate the turbulent waters of a breast cancer diagnosis if you have to, and navigate more peacefully through the rest of your life if you don't.

Let's begin. ❧

7

Take a Deep Breath

Our breath is the simplest and one of the most effective tools we have to counteract stress. At some point, we've all been advised to "Take a deep breath" when we were out of sorts and in danger of doing something we might later regret. There is deep physiologic truth in this advice. In the battle to counteract stress, the breath is a powerful, yet often overlooked, asset. The breath has a more profound effect on our health than most realize. What you *don't* know about it may surprise you.

Unique Features of the Breath

Breath is basic to life; we all know that. We can do without food for a month or so, without water for up to a week, but we can't survive without air for more than a few minutes. Most of what Western science knows about the breath is limited to the physiology of gas exchange. But there's so much more to it than that.

The role breath plays in maintaining homeostasis, for instance, is often overlooked. Most of us think of our bowels or bladder when we think of the elimination of waste products, but 70% of the body's waste products are eliminated through the lungs.[1] The physiologic effect of each breath is relatively small, but because we take over 20,000 breaths a day, the cumulative effect is greater than we realize.

Anything that affects our metabolism affects the breath. The increased metabolic demands of the stress response cause our breathing to become more rapid, allowing for greater gas exchange. When we are relaxed, our metabolic needs are less, so our breathing slows. Thus, **our breathing pattern is an accurate, moment-to-moment reflection of our internal state—a direct window into our physiology.**

There are two main types of breathing: Abdominal Breathing (also known as Belly Breathing) and Chest Breathing.[2] Which one predominates depends on what's going on with our physiology at the moment.

When we are relaxed, we breathe abdominally. This is the way we breathe when we are asleep. It's also how infants breathe. In this type of breathing, the abdomen is relaxed on the inhale allowing the diaphragm to descend as far as possible. This allows for maximal expansion of the lungs.

This is the most efficient type of breath because it brings more air into the bases of the lungs where blood supply is greatest. Abdominal breathing also affects the vagus nerve (a major trunk of the parasympathetic nervous system) as it passes through the opening in the central portion of the diaphragm. When stimulated, it calms us down. The deeper the breath, the more relaxed we become.

When we're stressed, we breathe mostly from the chest. Air is drawn in by expansion and contraction of the intercostal muscles (the muscles between the ribs) rather than by the action of the more efficient diaphragm. Chest Breathing is shallower than the deeper, more relaxed abdominal breath, and because it does not deliver the same amount of oxygen to the body per breath, we must breathe more rapidly to make up the difference.

Take a Deep Breath

Not only does our level of stress correspond to a particular breathing pattern, but so do our varied emotional states. When we're sad, we sigh; breathing in normally and breathing out more forcefully. When we're surprised, we gasp; breathing in quickly and forcefully, pausing on the inbreath. Beautiful sights, especially unexpected ones, are said to "take our breath away." Each human emotion has its unique signature on the breath. We can deny our feelings with our words, but our breath will always give us away.

Even our brain waves, a measure of the electrical activity of the brain, affect our breathing patterns.[3] When we're relaxed, the electrical activity of the brain is characterized by low frequency waves called alpha waves. When we're anxious, higher frequency beta waves predominate.

In the so-called alpha state, characterized by deep relaxation, increased awareness and high levels of creativity, we breathe slower, deeper, and abdominally. We breathe shallower and more rapidly when beta waves predominate.

All of these functions—brain wave activity, emotions, our state of arousal, and the breath—work automatically. They are under the control of the autonomic nervous system (ANS), which means they work without our having to think about them.

As opposed to the other functions, however, **the breath is under both conscious *and* unconscious control.** We're free to breathe however we like. We can breathe deeply one breath and shallow the next, or not breathe at all, at least for a minute or two. Or we can forget about our breath altogether and trust it to sustain us without paying any attention to it at all. It can be under voluntary control, or completely on automatic. Nothing in the human body is like it.

This makes perfect sense from a survival standpoint. If we refuse to eat or drink, we will eventually die. But we can't refuse to breathe indefinitely. We can hold our breath until we turn blue if we want, but after we pass out we'll always wake up to find ourselves breathing again. In terms of the breath, at least, if our conscious mind decides to do something foolish, the automatic system comes to the rescue.

The central nervous system (CNS) regulates our interactions with the outside world. It allows us to have voluntary control over certain functions. It is our ability to consciously control the breath that allows us to communicate verbally. Without it, the spoken word would be impossible. The ANS on the other hand, maintains our internal environment. It regulates heart rate, blood pressure, and the other functions that keep us alive. The breath, being the only function in the body under the influence of both, acts as a bridge between the two.

Modern medicine is well aware of the link between the breath and our internal physiologic state. Many conditions, particularly metabolic disorders, are associated with typical breathing patterns. Part of every medical school curriculum is devoted to teaching these patterns.

What modern medicine is not so well aware of is that **the intimate connection between our breath and our physiology is *a two-way street*.** It is a reciprocal relationship. Our level of stress affects our breath, but how we breathe affects our level of stress. Our emotional state affects our breathing pattern, but our breathing pattern also affects our emotional state.

Even our brain waves are affected by the pattern of our breathing. We can change both our state of arousal and our level of awareness simply by how we choose to breathe. If our breathing has the power to change even the electrical activity of our brain, what bodily process does it *not* affect? The answer, of course, is none. The breath affects everything.

It is this reciprocal relationship, the two-way street between our breathing and physiology, coupled with the fact that we can consciously choose how we breathe, that makes the breath not only a useful diagnostic tool, but a therapeutic one as well. The breath is both an indicator *and* a regulator of our physiology. It gives us a connection to *and* a degree of control over our internal environment—and therefore our health.

The Breath in Modern Medicine

Modern medicine does make use of these unique features of the breath, but only on a limited level. Critical care physicians use these principles every day to manage their ventilator patients in the intensive care unit (ICU). Ventilator settings are carefully monitored in terms of the volume of air delivered per breath and the number of breaths per minute, with predictable effects on the patient's physiology. This is as integral a part of managing a ventilator patient as any drug.

The use of the breath to control pain during childbirth is also well-accepted practice. Lamaze classes became popular more than thirty years ago, and have remained so ever since, because the breathing techniques they teach work. Every obstetrician I know encourages their patients to use them. It gives the mother-to-be a degree of control, and makes the delivering doctor's job easier.

Of course, the same breathing patterns used to control pain during childbirth would be just as useful in dealing with pain from any cause. And tailored breathing exercises would be useful in managing medical conditions before a patient is sick enough to be in the ICU. But outside of the ICU and delivery room, using the breath to alleviate pain, decrease stress, or to effect internal physiologic change, is almost unheard of. With very few exceptions, it's outside the medical paradigm.

Chapter Seven

Luckily, working with the breath is simple, and anyone can do it. Basically, it all comes down to this: by consciously choosing a relaxed breathing pattern, your body will follow suit, with all the attendant physical and mental benefits. If you're feeling anxious—for any reason—simply slowing down your breathing will diminish your anxiety. And it will do so 100 percent of the time.

Not all of us can think happy thoughts when we're stressed, but anyone can breathe slower. A relaxed breath will help see you through any crisis. And a consistently relaxed breath will bring your physiology into balance, decreasing your risk of chronic disease.

Breath truly is a miracle. Yes, it keeps us alive, but there's so much more to it than that. As a bridge between our conscious mind and our physiology, it gives us more control over our thoughts, emotions, and physical health than we ever thought possible. No wonder Andrew Weil calls it "The Master Key to Health." But as powerful a tool as it can be physiologically, there are deeper levels to this mysterious thing we call breath.

Breath as Metaphor

Breath can be seen as a metaphor for the rhythms of life. The never ending cycle of our breath—in and out, in and out, in and out for a lifetime—serves as a mirror of all creation. The tides ebb and flow; day follows night, which follows day; seasons come and go, and come again. Many scientists believe the entire universe, which is presently expanding, will someday begin to contract, and then expand again. The universe itself may be breathing—with a rhythm all its own.

The breath is a symbol of perfect balance. No human life has ever had an uneven number of inhalations and exhalations. All of us enter the world on an inbreath, and each of us leaves on an outbreath, a fact so unalterable that Western medicine uses the term "expired" as a euphemism for death.

A Symbol of Our Interconnectedness

With each breath, we exchange trillions of atoms with the environment.[4] This means that in a single exhale, trillions of atoms that used to be part of our bodies no longer are, and on the next inhale, we acquire trillions more.

What happens to all those atoms after we bid them farewell? Anything and everything. Some are inhaled by our neighbors and become part of them. Some are eagerly breathed in by the plants. The animals that eat the plants then get some of them. And if we happen to eat one of those animals, we will eventually get some of them back.

It's a disconcerting thought, but when you sit down to dinner with friends, by the time the evening is finished, each of you will go home "owning" a fair number of atoms that began the night belonging to someone else. No one owns them, of course. When it comes to our physical building blocks, we're all just renting.

How extensive is this exchange? In time it is complete. Over roughly a seven-year period, every atom in your body is completely replaced. Where do they go? Everywhere. They transfer indiscriminately to other humans, animals, plants and inanimate objects alike. Molecularly speaking, there is no difference between the carbon in your body and the carbon in this page. They are completely interchangeable.

Our bodies may look solid and separate, but they're not. They are in constant flux with the environment. If you could watch a time-lapse movie of what happens to the molecules of every living thing on the planet, you'd be able to see this free exchange. We are more like different currents in the same ocean than we are discrete and separate entities.

Why is this important? Because this insight carries the potential to change the way we think about others, our environment, and ourselves. When you can look at the person next to you and realize that in a very real sense they *are* you, everything changes. Compassion is a lot easier to come by when you realize we're all living the same life through different eyes.

It is also more difficult to treat the environment casually once we understand it as an extension of ourselves. Our relationship to the world we live in is much more fluid than we previously thought. Some even call the earth our "extended body." This should make us think twice before we disregard the environment. When it suffers, to some degree we all suffer.

Deeper Questions

Understanding the depth of our interconnectedness challenges some of our most basic assumptions about disease. If each atom in our body turns over every seven years, how can we have the same chronic injuries and diseases we've had for decades? Why do some of the new building blocks form cancer cells, some degenerated discs, and some completely healthy cells? Why don't the cells all form like new? There's nothing wrong with the building blocks.

Eastern medical practices are based on the premise that there is an energy field that provides a template upon which the human (or any other) body is formed. From this point of view, disease arises as a disturbance in the field long before it manifests in the physical body. The fact that you can live with a diseased organ for thirty years, even though every cell in that organ has been replaced multiple times, with perfectly good building blocks, would seem to substantiate this view.

Western theologians might call this energy field the human spirit, and their view that all disease has a spiritual origin is not dissimilar to Eastern medical philosophy, which approaches disease from an energetic standpoint.

It may seem like we're far afield from our original discussion. But these deeper considerations are exactly where the cancer journey leads if we can break through our fears long enough to ask the questions. We fear cancer because it threatens to end our earthly existence, but what is the real nature of this earthly existence? And why are we so afraid of losing it?

Breath and Spirit

Many cultures consider Spirit and breath one and the same. Many languages have only one word to describe them both:[5]

Sanskrit	*prana*
Chinese	*chi*
Hebrew	*ruach*
Greek	*pneuma*
Latin	*spiritus*

To distinguish it from the physical process of breathing, Hindu sages often refer to the *pranic* life force as "the Breath behind the breath." Spiritual masters in China do much the same, referring to the physical breath as the "outer breath," and divine life force, *chi,* as the "Inner Breath."

The dual meaning of the Hebrew word *ruach* is responsible for the different appearance of some verses in various Bible translations. Ancient Hebrew scribes often paired the word *ruach* with *Yahweh,* the name of the God of Israel. But *ruach Yahweh* can be translated as "the breath of God," the "spirit of God," or even "the wind of God" (God's breath manifest as the wind), depending on the meaning given to *ruach*.

In the Western world, the connection between breath and Spirit has been lost, but it remains deeply rooted in our language. Our word inspiration, derived from the Latin *spiritus*, can mean that we are influenced by the divine, or might only refer to the physical act of drawing in air.

The connection is preserved in our language, but not in our everyday awareness. Somehow we've lost track. Andy Caponigro, author of *The Miracle of the Breath*, considers this "one of the most unfortunate blind spots in Western thinking," and believes we have "overlooked a spiritual Rosetta stone that can help us decipher some of the deepest mysteries of human existence...."

Is the Spirit of God and the physical breath really one and the same, or is it just a metaphor? We can never know for sure, but it would be just like God to hide himself right under our noses.

Working with the Breath

The breath is a paradox. It's so simple we don't have to think about it, yet there are entire books written on the subject. Some spend their entire lives trying to master it, while others never think about it at all. If you're interested in learning about the breath in more detail, Caponigro's The Miracle of the Breath is a good place to start. It is a comprehensive, easy-to-read, and fascinating introduction to the breath, written in a style that's easy for Westerners to take in.

Because our immediate focus is stress reduction, however, I'd like to end the chapter on a practical note. Simply put, the breath is the number one tool to reach for when you feel out of sorts.

Take a Deep Breath

Nothing else will so quickly, easily, and reliably calm you down. It is medicine in every sense of the word.

The following are two techniques of working with the breath. There are hundreds of others, but for reducing stress, these are the most basic.

Take a deep breath. This is your "911" tool for stress. Use it any time you feel anxious, for any reason. If you're by yourself, inhale through the nose and let the air out forcefully through your mouth with a *whoosh* sound. You can enhance the effect by raising you arms overhead with fists clenched on the inhale, then bringing them quickly to your sides and spreading your fingers on the exhale. Do this in a throwing motion, as if you were casting your anxiety into the ground.

If you're in public, and want to keep your reputation intact, let the air out less forcefully, but still more accentuated than the inhale, and you can skip the arm motions. Remember, we do this automatically when we sigh. It's how our bodies discharge emotional energy. You can do the same thing consciously to enhance the physiologic effect. Think of it as a "purposeful sigh." Repeat the pattern until your anxiety starts to diminish.

Focus on breathing deeper, slower, quieter, and more rhythmic.[6] Once you're feeling calmer, shift into this pattern. Or if your anxiety is mild, you can start here. You can do this anywhere; no one will notice. It can also be done as a relaxation practice even when you're not feeling anxious. Done as a regular practice, it can retrain the breath, returning it to a more balanced pattern. This can have untold benefits for your health. Remember: deeper.....slower.....quieter.....and more rhythmic..... ∂

8
Making Meditation
Your Friend

જે

When we think of meditation, most of us get a mental picture of a yogi sitting on a pillow in the lotus position chanting "Om." While this is meditation, it is only one particular type and one particular style, out of hundreds or thousands. The biggest obstacle to meditation is our preconceived notion that we already know what it is.

Meditation is broader in scope than most think. The Eastern-style sitting meditation is no more representative of the entirety of meditation than socks are representative of clothing. It is only part of a very large whole.

Meditation is not Eastern or Western—it just is. Every spiritual and religious tradition has meditative practices, but meditation is not religious in itself. It is a basic human capacity. The best way to consider meditation is to strip away the cultural and religious connotations, break it down to its lowest common denominator, and see how it affects human physiology. Once you understand its essence, you can then take the basics and build them into a practice that makes sense to you.

The wide range of practices that qualify as meditation may surprise you. In fact, we've already talked about meditation; we just didn't call it that. Focusing on the breath is one of the oldest and most powerful types of meditation. But there are so many more.

A Definition

Like stress, meditation can be difficult to define. In the broadest sense, meditation is a moment-to-moment awareness, a quieting of the mind which brings us into the "here and now." It is often defined as focused awareness, but it can also be a letting go of all focus, leading to a more expansive awareness.

Some have defined awareness as "perception without judgment." Of the two parts of this definition, it's the "without judgment" that's the key. If we have difficulty with any part of meditation, this is usually the part. Most of us judge far more than we know. Judgment is more than bigotry or criticism. We make snap judgments about people and situations all the time.

The stories about Bill, Mary, and Jim in chapter six were judgments. Our Inner Storyteller is far more active than we realize. It is constantly telling us "how things are"—even though quite often that's *not* how they are. Judgments are inherently stressful. And they're self-inflicted. Meditation helps us become aware of them.

Meditation is about having no notions at all, preconceived or otherwise. It's about noticing, and nothing else. Don't judge. Don't analyze. Just notice. This is the "work" of meditation. This is difficult for most of us because reasoning and analysis are so highly regarded in our culture. And then there's that darned Storyteller.

Types of Meditation

James S. Gordon, M.D., Founder and Director of the Center for Mind-Body Medicine, breaks down the many different styles of meditation into three basic types:

1. **Concentrative meditation** involves focusing our awareness on a particular object, which might be an image, a word, or even a sound. Focusing on the breath is a type of concentrative meditation. Prayer is also considered a type of concentrative meditation.

2. **Awareness mediation,** also known as mindfulness meditation, involves no specific point of focus. It is simply being relaxed and aware of thoughts, feelings, and sensations as they arise. This is the "simply noticing" type of meditation. Sometimes it involves being aware of bodily sensations. Sometimes it's just observing your own thoughts as they arise.

3. **Moving meditation** is the oldest type of meditation. Shaking, dancing, some types of rhythmic breathing and yoga are examples of moving mediations. Also called expressive meditations, these are seldom thought of as meditation, but are just as powerful as the more sedentary types, sometimes more so.

Physical Benefits

The word meditation is derived from the Latin *medicus,* which means "to take the measure of," or "to care for." This is the same Latin root from which our word medicine is derived. This seems appropriate considering the many and varied health benefits of meditation. Meditation is at the heart of all healing. It is the cornerstone of self-care—the centerpiece of mind-body medicine.

Of all the mind-body skills, meditation has been the most thoroughly studied by Western science. Herbert Benson, M.D., a pioneer in mind-body medicine and well known for his research on stress, did the first extensive studies in the West on Transcendental

Chapter Eight

Meditation (TM) at Harvard Medical School. TM is a concentrative meditation that involves repeating a single word or phrase, called a "mantra," over and over. The word "mantra" comes from two different Sanskrit roots which, when used together, mean *mind tool*. This is how the repetitive word or phrase functions during meditation—as a tool to fix the attention.

Benson discovered that the physiologic response to meditation is predictable and reproducible. Blood pressure, pulse, and respiratory rate decrease, blood is shunted away from the large muscles, and so on, all being mediated by the parasympathetic nervous system. In short, meditation relaxes us.

It was Benson who coined the phrase "relaxation response" for these physiologic changes to underscore the fact that they counteract the fight or flight response.[1] Meditation has its greatest healing effects by balancing the sympathetic overload so common to Western culture.

It is important to note that the physiologic benefits of meditation occur not only while you are actively meditating, but continue even when you're not. If you meditate fifteen minutes a day, most of the beneficial effects are taking place in the other twenty-three hours and forty-five minutes.

Long-term meditators have:[2,3,4]

- Lower blood pressure
- Lower resting pulse
- Lower levels of cortisol and adrenaline
- Lower blood sugar
- Enhanced immunity
- Reduced biological age

Because of the ongoing physiologic benefits, meditation can have a dramatic effect on illnesses that result from a stressful lifestyle.

Meditation reduces the risk of chronic disease, decreases the side effects of therapy and improves quality of life in cancer patients, and raises the pain threshold.[5,6,7] Meditative techniques, in conjunction with other mind-body skills, have even prolonged survival in breast cancer patients.[8]

Mental Benefits

In the sense that we have to pay attention to something, we're actually meditating all the time. Unfortunately, we mostly pay attention to our thoughts as they're racing to and fro. We don't recognize this as meditation because of the scattered nature of the thoughts. It is estimated we have between 40,000 to 60,000 thoughts a day, most of them repetitive, and a large percentage of them negative.

In meditative circles this has been called "puppy mind" because the untrained mind is similar to that of a puppy that can't go from here to the driveway without chasing every bee and butterfly in sight. It is also known as "monkey mind" because of a monkey's tendency to scurry endlessly from one branch to the next. These colorful metaphors point to one of the fundamental problems of modern culture—the untrained mind can't fix its attention on anything for long.

When our attention follows our mental chatter, we don't recognize the power of our attention. We experience its power only when we focus. It's much like the difference between a light bulb and a laser beam. The light from the bulb is scattered in all directions. It provides enough light for us to see, but not much more than that. A laser, on the other hand, is a beam of *focused* light. For the same wattage, the power of a laser is exponentially greater.

By increasing our ability to focus, meditation brings out the innate power of the human mind—power that's been diffused by our mental chatter for so long we've forgotten it exists. Herbert Benson's work proves it exists, and that this power is available to all of us.

Meditation is mental training. It's taking our mind to the gym and working it out. Let's face it—most of us are mental couch potatoes. There's no work we shrink from more than mental work. No one ever told us it was important. No one ever showed us how to do it. But it *is* important, and once you get the hang of it, it's not that hard.

Meditation:

- Enhances our ability to focus
- Slows the mental chatter
- Increases self-awareness
- Brings us into the present moment
- Helps us recognize stressful thought patterns
- Enhances mental clarity
- Changes brain wave patterns

Meditation enhances every mental capacity. It enlarges our perspective, allowing us to see the world and ourselves more clearly, less judgmentally, and with more compassion. It is one of the most potent tools we have for taking care of ourselves.

By quieting our mental chatter, meditation brings us stillness. And in stillness, there is peace. Peace doesn't mean being in a place where there is no noise, trouble, or hard work. It means to be in the midst of those things and still be calm in our heart. The ability to keep our peace in the face of whatever life throws at us is one of the great gifts of meditation.

Presence

The moment-to-moment awareness of meditation leads quite naturally to a discussion of presence. Like meditation and stress, presence can be difficult to put into words. Living in the present moment with our full attention may be the closest one can come to a definition. On the surface this seems simple, but it's harder than you might think. Physically, it's easy—you can't actually be anyplace other than where you are. But mentally, it's a different story.

So often, when we're at work, we're thinking about home, and when we're home, we're thinking about work. When we're driving, we think about where we're going or where we've been. Rarely do we give our full attention to what we're doing right now. It gets *some* of our attention, but rarely does it get all of it.

Feeling overwhelmed by all we have to do is a classic example of not being fully present. No matter how much we have to do, it's only possible to do one thing at a time. Regardless of how long the list is, the one thing can always be done in peace—as long as we focus only on the one thing. Feeling overwhelmed is a result of mentally trying to do all of them at once.

What does this have to do with breast cancer? In a word, stress. Being physically here, but mentally there, is inherently stressful. It is an internal pulling apart, which is the very definition of stress. The "don't-have-enough-time," and "have-to-get-it-all-done-now" syndromes will, over time, degrade the immune system and increase our risk of chronic disease.

There's always enough time to do everything you need to get done. There's not always enough time to do everything you *want* to get done. Knowing the difference can be a lifesaver. Some people refer to time urgency as "hurry sickness," which is more than just a metaphor. Time urgency is a major risk factor for heart disease and hypertension, though an association with cancer risk is still unclear.[9,10]

Presence is about being content with whatever we're doing in the moment, without regard to what will come of it. It's about not making this moment a stepping-stone to the next. Most of us wash the dishes, for instance, so we can have a clean kitchen. There's nothing wrong with that; one necessarily leads to the other. But when we consider the washing less important than having them done, we sacrifice the present for the future. This is the "I'll be happy when…" mentality so many of us fall prey to. When we habitually look at life this way, we end up wishing away a large part of it.

Each moment of life is equally important. There are no small moments. If you're washing the dishes—wash the dishes. If you have to do them anyway, you might as well enjoy it. And if you're going to be there physically, you might as well be there mentally too. Notice how the water feels on your hands. Notice the pattern on the plates. Be thankful you have running water. Don't do them just to get them done. Do them because this is your chosen task in life at this moment—your only task.

Doing the dishes in this manner can be a metaphor for life. If you pay full attention, doing the small things with excellence for their own sake, the big things will take care of themselves. Anything you do with presence will shine. Others may not know *why* it shines, but they'll notice the shine. Presence isn't about what you do; it's about how you do it. All of life is about how you do it.

Meditation and Spirit

It's in presence that meditation begins to blend with Spirit. Eternity is made up of an endless number of present moments. Tomorrow never comes; it's always today. The future and the past are psychological entities. They provide a way for us to catalog events as they occur in the material realm, but they have no meaning outside the human mind. It's always now. It can't be anything else.

The present moment is sometimes referred to as the Sacred Now because it's the only place we can meet God. In fact, it *is* God. When Moses inquired about God's name, God replied, "I Am." This is the nature of God—pure Being. God is everywhere, which means God is always fully present. When we are fully present, our nature matches divine nature. Our "I am" merges with *the* "I Am," and magic happens. It is Holy Communion in every sense.

The Aborigines refer to God as "Divine Oneness," which is a wonderful description of the omnipresence of Universal Intelligence. It is everywhere. And if we're paying attention, we can perceive it in everything. It's always available to us. The only question is—are we available to it? The Brothers Frantzich put it this way in a song: "God will not be present unless we are."[11]

Meditative practices are part of every religion, and even though some Christian groups teach against it, there is a rich history of meditation in Christianity. Prayer itself is a type of meditation. Father Thomas Keating, a well-known Catholic writer, says "For me, meditation is non-conceptual prayer, a relationship with God that emphasizes the heart rather than the mind."

Quieting the mind before prayer is like taking your muddy shoes off before walking into your living room. God isn't going to yell at you if you don't, but the ethereal realm is so subtle you won't be able to connect well. There is deep physiologic truth in the verse, "Be still and know I am God" (Psalm 46:10). Spiritual experiences occur more commonly in the lower frequency brain wave states, which is exactly where meditation takes you.

The corollary to this verse (my invention) is equally true: "If you *aren't* still, you *won't* know I am God." God will still be God, of course—he can't be anything else. But the mental chatter of the higher frequency brain wave states will drown out your ability to perceive him. Without a quiet mind, your awareness will be stuck in the everyday, not the eternal.

There are dozens of verses relating to meditation in both the Old and New Testaments. "I have calmed and quieted my soul, like a weaned child," David said in Psalm 131. Why did he do this? Because he couldn't hear his Beloved if he didn't.

One of the best descriptions of a mantra can be found in the words of an influential but unknown Christian mystic who wrote *The Cloud of Unknowing* sometime during the middle ages. In a section entitled, "How a person should conduct himself during prayer with regard to all thoughts," he writes:[12]

> It is inevitable that ideas will arise in your mind and try to distract you in a thousand ways…before you know it, your mind is completely scattered…gather all your desire into one simple word that the mind can easily retain…A one-syllable word such as "God" or "love" is best. But choose one that is meaningful to you. Then fix it in your mind so that it will remain there come what may. This word will be your defense in conflict and in peace. Use it to… subdue all distractions….Should some thought go on annoying you demanding to know what you are doing, answer with this one word alone….Do this and I assure you these thoughts will vanish.

A Word about Words

For many in the West, the words "meditation" and "mantra" carry an emotional charge. These words have Eastern connotations, and for some they are considered taboo. No one has a problem with the words "medicine" or "mind," however, even though they are derived from the same Sanskrit roots. This makes it clear that the emotional charge is due to our perspective—not the words themselves.

Making Meditation Your Friend

The emotional charge we feel from certain words is the result of a judgment or a preconceived notion. Sometimes we develop these ourselves, associating a particular word with a past unpleasant event. Just as often, we absorb them unconsciously from our parents or a cultural or religious paradigm. But regardless of what we think about them, words are just words.

Language is a tool, nothing more. Words are written symbols or uttered sounds that convey a deeper meaning. No group owns a word, no matter how often they might use it. There is a Buddhist saying, "The finger pointing to the moon is not the moon." Words are merely fingers; it's best not to get hung up on them. It's the moon we're after.

Our prejudices act like an invisible fence for pets. As long as the fence is "charged" we will never investigate what's on the other side. In our case, unlike the pet, the barrier is self-imposed, the charge being supplied by our own judgments. There is often great truth to be found beyond the fence, but if we can't get past our judgments, we will never find it. Ultimately, this is what our judgments do—separate us from others.

Once we let go of our judgments, life can be surprising. I remember when I wouldn't pick up a book like this, and now I find myself writing one. It's amazing what can happen when our self-imposed fences disappear.

My advice on the subject is this: if the word "meditation" offends you, call it something else. Tom Kenyon, in his book *Brain States*, calls it "regular systemic stabilization," because physiologically that's what it is. The same goes for the word "mantra." If it puts you off in any way, call it a "mind anchor," or better still, just use it and don't call it anything at all.

If for you, meditation is prayer, then pray. If you think of it more as routine mental and physical maintenance, then do your routine maintenance. If for you, it's sitting in the lotus position chanting "Om," then sit in the lotus position and chant "Om." Do what works for you, and more importantly, let everyone else do the same.

The terms "meditation," "prayer," "regular systemic stabilization," and "relaxation response," are different doors to the same storehouse. If any of these say "Keep Out" to you, use a different door; don't miss out altogether. The material in the storehouse is too valuable.

The power of the human mind is available to everyone. Don't avoid the subject because people who seem different than you are taking advantage of it. Use it yourself in your own way. If you stick with it, meditation will eventually show you that "those people" are no different than you.

My Favorite Kinds of Meditation

The following is a list of my favorite meditations. Interestingly, I never considered most of them meditation. Only after I understood what meditation was did I realize how much I was meditating.

Writing: Not surprisingly, I find writing meditative. Probably because it slows down the mind. Thoughts are fleeting, but committing them to paper requires us to dwell on them longer than we would otherwise. This may be why journaling is so powerful. My writing career began as simple journaling. I never thought of being published—I just did it for *me*.

Contemplative prayer: Simply adding an intention to connect with God changes a sitting meditation into contemplative prayer, something I find endlessly interesting and profoundly moving. It's been said that prayer is talking to God and meditation is listening to God. It works for me. Sometimes I don't know what to say anyway.

Making Meditation Your Friend

Being in nature: All of nature is completely present. As far as we know, trees and flowers don't worry about the next drought, and birds aren't concerned about tomorrow's breakfast. When we connect with nature, we are drawn into its immense presence. The beauty and wonder of nature can bring us back to our own nature— if we allow it.

Being around children or animals: Children and animals are more innocent than we are—and not nearly as complicated. It's easier to be in touch with that part of myself when I'm around them. It's been said that if you want to experience unconditional love, don't get married, buy a dog. While it's true that a committed adult relationship can be a thing of joy—the dog *is* a lot simpler.

Biking: Any sport can be meditative because they all require focus. Sport can be a great respite for the obsessive mind. I find biking particularly meditative. I'm out in nature, I'm locked into the pedals, so I can't go anywhere the bike doesn't go, and the constant cadence of the pedals is soothing to the mind. It's an automatic mantra that continues in the background no matter how far I go.

Photography: Looking at life through a camera lens allows me to see it differently. I appreciate the wonder more. I see the beauty that's so easy to miss when I'm walking down the street lost in thought. Not surprisingly, nature and animal photography are my favorites.

Breathwork: What I do can't be called breath*work*, exactly. It's more like breath play. I do a few basic breathing exercises, but mostly I just experiment. I find the breath interesting and fun. I have it with me wherever I go and the possibilities are nearly endless. It doesn't matter what I do with my breath; as long as I'm paying attention to it, I'm meditating. How easy is that?

Yoga: Nothing will keep you looking and feeling younger than yoga. I love the combination of exercise, breathing, and focus. And no, it isn't a religion. It is a prescribed set of postures linked to the breath—a moving meditation. It isn't a religion any more than the Waltz or the Tango. You can make it one if you wish, and some do, but there's nothing inherently religious about the postures.

Sitting meditations: My favorite sitting meditations are practices I call allowing and labeling. To begin the *allowing practice,* sit quietly for a few minutes, focusing on your breath or another mental anchor. When thoughts come to mind, as they inevitably will, allow whatever comes up to be perfect just as it is.

Difficult situations are what usually come to mind, of course. In life we tend to worry about them, avoid them, or otherwise resist them. But in this practice, the goal is to accept them just as they are. To make peace with them without wishing things were different. This practice doesn't change the situations, but it changes us—which is effectively the same thing.

Sometimes I repeat the phrase "It's okay," softly to myself, to remind me that any situation can be okay in my quiet time, even if I don't think so in real life. When we mentally accept situations as they are, stress drops away quickly. I'm often surprised by how gentle and soothing the "It's okay" feels. Sometimes it sounds like a loving parent comforting an anxious child, which on some level I'm sure it is.

Labeling practice begins the same way as allowing practice, by focusing on the breath or other mental anchor until you are relaxed. In this practice, however, when thoughts come, you simply label them: "Worried about the bills," "Angry at my boss," "Don't like my kids' friends," and so on.

In real life when we have these thoughts, we consider the bills, the boss, and the kids' friends the problem. But in this meditation we don't judge our thoughts as either true or false. We simply label them, let them go, and wait for the next one to appear.

You can learn a lot about yourself by cataloging your thoughts without getting lost in the story the thoughts are trying to tell you. Meditation makes us less gullible to our own stories, giving us more control over our lives.

I love the allowing and labeling practices because they bypass one of the common mistakes made by beginners—trying to forcefully quiet the mind. Thoughts aren't the enemy. Minds think. That's what they do. Trying to bully the mind into being quiet sets up a cycle of inner conflict. It's your ego shaming your ego for acting like an ego—a no-win situation if there ever was one.

The biggest enemies of meditation are self-judgment and expectations. These make meditation seem difficult by telling us two things: We *should* be doing it better and things *should* be different. Once we begin to just notice the "shoulds," without necessarily believing what they tell us, meditation becomes a lot easier. Our thoughts and judgments then become the very things that make meditation so rich. It doesn't matter what we're observing—as long as we're just observing.

A Few Final Words

When someone asked well-known yoga teacher David Williams during a yoga retreat if he meditated, he answered, "When I lose my meditation, then I go sit in the corner, if that's what you mean." Williams' statement shows us that even among people who meditate, meditation is often misunderstood.

Meditation is a way of life, not something you do fifteen minutes a day. Sitting quietly fifteen minutes a day might be the anchor of your practice, but ultimately, life is your meditation practice. You can work meditatively, drive meditatively, make love meditatively, or mow the lawn meditatively. But they are meditative only if you do them with your full attention. If you try to do more than one at the same time, *none* of them is meditative—and your lawn probably won't look so great either.

You can even eat meditatively, though few of us slow down enough to do it. What we eat is important, but it's just as important to pay attention to *why* we're eating it, *how* we're eating it, and how it affects our bodies. It's been said that how we eat is how we do life. If true, it explains a lot.

Many people don't meditate because they find it difficult. But meditation isn't difficult—our minds are difficult. Getting to know our own mind is work, but it's wonderful work with incredible benefits. Bernie Siegel, M.D., author of *Love, Medicine, and Miracles*, sums up the power of meditation by saying, "I know of no other single activity that by itself can produce such a great improvement in the quality of life."

Meditative practices are like shock absorbers and air bags for your life. They help you get over the bumps in the road easier, and soften the harder blows, making them more survivable. Every vehicle should have them, including human ones. The good news is that they're effective and they're free. The bad news is that you have to install them yourself.

Exercises

Make a list of your own favorite meditative practices. Formalize your list by committing it to paper. Use my list as a guide if you like. Don't judge an activity by what it is, only by how it makes you feel. Remember, meditation is about your internal physiologic state, not how you get there.

Read the rest of the book as a meditation. Evaluate your mental and emotional state and your level of receptivity each time you sit down to read. Read with your full attention for as long as the material holds your attention. Then do something else with your full attention.

Consider the whole book an exercise. Take your time. Remember, this is "taking-a-bubble-bath-with-a-glass-of-wine" kind of reading not the "take-a-shower-and-rush-off-to-work" kind. Consider the deeper implications of each section. If you skim the surface, you will be limited to the information on the page. If you take time to go deeper, you'll get so much more than that. ❧

9

The Power of Imagination

೭

We will begin this chapter with a brief exercise called a guided imagery. Read through it slowly, closing your eyes periodically to allow the images to develop fully. This will be your first practice at reading meditatively. Take as much time as you need.

This exercise has to do with the images in your mind. The words are only there to guide you. Stay with the images as long as they keep developing. Come back to the words when you need to.

*I'd like you to imagine that you're standing in your kitchen......
Take a few moments to notice all the details......See it in
color......the tiles on the floor......the appliances......the countertops......Take your time, allowing the images to become as
vivid as possible......Use all your senses. Maybe you can hear
the hum of the refrigerator, or the ticking of the clock on the
wall......Notice what you smell......maybe there's something
baking in the oven......Notice what you're wearing....how you
feel.....whether it's daytime or night........*

*Looking down at one of the countertops, notice a cutting
board with a lemon sitting on it and a sharp knife beside
it......Don't let the details be fuzzy. See a specific countertop, a
specific cutting board, and a specific knife..........Pick up the*

Chapter Nine

lemon.......Notice the weight......the size......the color.......feel the texture and moisture on the outside of the peel......Now put it back on the cutting board, pick up the knife and cut it in half......Notice the juice as it runs out onto the cutting board along with a few seeds......

Now take one of the halves, and cut a wedge out of it......Pick up the lemon wedge......Bring it to your nose and smell the freshness of it......Then put it in your mouth and bite into the soft, juicy pulp.........

[with permission. James S. Gordon, M.D., Center for Mind-Body Medicine]

How many ways did your body respond to the imagery? Could you see it, feel it, taste it? You may have salivated when you bit down on the imaginary lemon. Depending on how vivid your images were, you may have contorted your face or even shivered a bit.

If you didn't salivate, or if you did and want to deepen the experience, put the book down, go into your kitchen, and look at everything you just imagined. Pay attention to the detail of the countertops. See how they feel. Hear the sounds. Smell the smells. Repeat the exercise in real life. You may even want to get a lemon out if you have one.

In doing this, you may notice more detail about your kitchen than you normally do. If so, it's because you are more present than usual—you're paying more attention. What you're doing is a mindfulness meditation on your kitchen. Notice how much more alive you feel compared to most of the time you spend there.

When you're ready, leave your kitchen and repeat the imagery. If you didn't salivate the first time it's likely you will after strengthening your mental images. It's a basic tenet of imagery that the more lifelike your mental images, the stronger the response.

The Power of Imagination

If you salivated either time, you've just experienced imagery's ability to trigger a physical response. You can read volumes of research on the mind-body connection, but what you just experienced proves one exists. Look around—there probably isn't a lemon in the room. There may not be one in the entire house. And yet, because you pictured one in your mind, your body reacted as if there were.

It is a well-established fact that our bodies cannot tell the difference between what is real and what is vividly imagined. Our mental images affect our physiology *directly* and *immediately*. You may have only been aware of the increase in saliva as you bit down on the imaginary lemon, but that's only the tip of the iceberg. A cascade of biochemical and hormonal changes took place, only part of which was the salivation. The physiologic response to our mental images is a whole-body response.

The Lemon Imagery makes it clear that this is more than just a philosophical discussion. Our bodies react to our mental images as if they were real events. Whether the images work to our benefit or to our detriment depends on the images. We didn't mention mental images in our earlier discussion on stress, but when we dwell on a disagreement with our boss or an argument with our spouse for weeks after the actual event, it's our mental images that are the issue, not what our boss or spouse did.

Our body reacts as if the event were still occurring because it's reacting to our mental images of the event, which are ongoing. It can't be reacting to the event itself, because the event is over and done with. Dwelling on unpleasant events from the past is a form of negative imagery, so-called because the images have a negative effect on our health. The most common form of imagery is worry, a form of negative imagery that focuses on possible future events.

Positive images can be as healing as negative ones are harmful.

Chapter Nine

This powerful effect can be seen in a study done in the 1970s by Dr. David Spiegel, a psychiatrist at Stanford University.[1] Spiegel divided eighty-six women with metastatic breast cancer into two groups. The first group received standard medical therapy and also took part in weekly group sessions for a year where they learned simple guided imagery. They were instructed to imagine themselves floating gently on water, feeling relaxed and peaceful, and encouraged to use this imagery whenever they were feeling stressed. The control group received standard medical therapy with no group sessions.

After one year, the first group reported a better quality of life, less pain and discomfort, and a greater feeling of control. The results were not unexpected, but what Spiegel discovered ten years later in reviewing the death records of both groups *was* unexpected. He found that the first group had survived an average of *twice* as long as the control group. Here was compelling evidence that the effects of mental imagery were at least partly responsible for not only improving quality of life, but increased survival as well.

For most of us, the process of imagery is a passive one. We think about whatever pops into our head, never realizing the immediate effect it has on our body. We worry when we're in the mood to worry, and we look forward to a bright future when our mood is more positive. But we also have the ability to create mental images. The images used by the participants in Spiegel's study were ones they created for themselves. Their ability to focus on these images consistently, crowding out stress-provoking images, clearly had a powerful healing effect.

Using imagery to improve our health involves learning to deal effectively with the resentments, worries, and regrets of everyday life, as well as creating specific healing images that are focused on regularly over a period of time. We all have the ability to do this. It is an integral part of the human design.

The Power of Imagination

Mental Images

The basis of all imagery is this: we think in pictures and not in words. If I ask you to think of an elephant, you will see a mental picture of an elephant and not the written word. If I asked you to think of a couch, an orange, or a grapefruit, it would be the same.

Mental pictures are said to be the original language of man. Written and spoken words are merely symbols of those images, developed to facilitate communication. Imagery isn't something we have to learn; we're already doing it. We need only become aware of it so we can consciously make it work for us.

One way to increase our awareness is to mentally slow things down. A meditation practice helps calm our minds, allowing us easier access to the stream of images underneath. Our minds work at an incredible speed. The typical state of our mental affairs is like driving a car on the highway. At ninety miles per hour we see the landscape out the window, but we lose a lot of the detail, and much of the beauty. It's easier to see both when we're traveling thirty miles per hour down a country road.

We may not be aware of our mental images, but they are always present. If we feel anxious or worried, we can be sure there are fearful images playing on our mental movie screens somewhere. If we're at peace, there are pleasant ones. Our conscious minds may not be aware of them, but our bodies are, and respond accordingly. Regaining conscious awareness of these images and learning to work with them constructively allows us to take control of our health and opens us to a world of wonder.

A Few Terms

Before going any further, it will be helpful to define a few terms.

Chapter Nine

The difference between visualization and imagery, for instance, is often misunderstood. **Visualization**, often described as "seeing with our mind's eye," refers specifically to mental pictures. **Imagery** refers not only to mental pictures, but also to auditory sensations, as well as those involving smell, taste, movement and touch. It can be a bit confusing since all visualization is imagery, but not all imagery is visualization.

For all intents and purposes, the two terms are interchangeable, keeping in mind that everything we experience mentally is not visual. It isn't the type of image that's important, but our physiologic response to it. Our bodies are just as responsive to auditory and tactile images as they are to visual ones. In fact, the more senses we involve in the process, the stronger the physiologic response will be.

The following is a brief description of the different categories and types of imagery. A more complete discussion can be found in Belleruth Naparstek's excellent book, *Staying Well with Guided Imagery*.

Receptive imagery refers to images that arise spontaneously. The images are always there, but they're usually below our level of conscious awareness. Experiencing receptive imagery, therefore, is mostly about getting into a relaxed state where we can more easily access them. Intuitive information comes by way of receptive imagery. Anyone can do this; it doesn't require a special gift.

Active imagery is the intentional use of images to help achieve a specific goal. This can be useful in virtually any area of life, from improving your golf swing, to increasing your monthly sales, to assisting in healing an illness. In active imagery the images are consciously created for a specific purpose.

Guided imagery is like a directed daydream. It is both active and receptive. Like the Lemon Imagery, it is directed from the outside, but the images are strictly our own. The process is guided from the outside, but not controlled from the outside.

Types of Imagery

There are many different types of imagery, all of which can fit into any of the three broad categories above. Perhaps the most basic, *emotional-state imagery,* is geared simply to changing your mood. Actors are very adept at this, using mental images to create whatever mood is appropriate for a particular scene. With practice, anyone can learn to change a bad mood to a good one by using mental images alone.

End-state imagery is another simple and effective type of imagery that involves imagining yourself already in the condition or circumstance that you wish for. This has also been called "mental rehearsal," where you see yourself as healthy, successful, cancer-free, and so on. As with emotional-state imagery, you don't need a lot of technical information. You just have to know what you want.

Imagery that involves physical processes in the body is called *physiological imagery.* This can even involve events in the body at the cellular level. We can use imagery to instruct immune cells to differentially attack some things and leave others alone, and those cells will follow suit. When people imagine their natural killer cells attacking and destroying cancer cells, there is a measurable increase in immune activity in the blood and saliva.[2] It sounds like science fiction, but it's scientific fact.

Physiological imagery can also be done on a more life-size scale, with focused mental pictures of arteries widening to provide increased blood flow to a specific area, or arteries narrowing to cut off blood supplying a tumor. Physiological imagery requires some technical knowledge, but this can easily be obtained by consulting your doctor, thumbing through a simple anatomy book, or looking online.

Metaphorical imagery is probably the most common type of imagery. Instead of anatomically correct images of natural killer cells attacking cancer cells, a person might imagine Pac-men scurrying around swallowing up alien intruders. This is just as effective as the more anatomically correct type. The possibilities are endless—limited only by our imagination.

Spiritual imagery is imagery that aims directly for connection with God. This might be in the form of images of, or even conversations with, God or great spiritual leaders. Spiritual imagery quite often takes the form of metaphor. Just because we're having an imaginary conversation with an animal, or a tree, or an inanimate object, doesn't mean it's not an interaction with the divine.

Like meditation, imagery has a negative connotation among some conservative religious groups. But many of those same groups use imagery as part of prayer; they just don't call it imagery. The boundary between imagery and prayer is a fuzzy one, if it exists at all. Belleruth Naparstek suggests that "perhaps all good prayer is a form of imagery, and all good imagery is a form of prayer."

Imagery is an interesting and diverse tool. None of the categories we've discussed is entirely distinct from the others. There are no fixed boundaries. Imagery is the crossroads between the material and the mystical. It is a place where worlds meet.

Regardless of type, imagery has tremendous healing potential as illustrated by the case of Glen, a young boy with an inoperable brain tumor described in Bernie Siegel's *Love, Medicine and Miracles*.[3] After Glen's doctor said further tests and treatments were useless and sent him home to die, his parents took him to the biofeedback center at the Mayo Clinic, where he learned imagery techniques.

Glen liked the idea of a rocket ship flying around in his head, shooting at the tumor, and he enjoyed blasting it regularly. After a few months he told his father, "I just took a trip through my head in the rocket ship and I can't find the cancer anymore." A follow-up CAT scan revealed no sign of the cancer.

It would be easy if it always worked this way, but it doesn't. We just don't know enough about the process to make it work this powerfully for everyone. But clearly the miraculous is possible. Complete healings are uncommon, but not unheard of. Improvement in quality of life and longer survival times in patients with advanced cancers are commonplace. If you have cancer and you're not making use of imagery, you're leaving a lot on the table.

History of Healing Imagery

Imagery is considered new to Western medicine, but it's been around for thousands of years. It was already well established by the time of the Greeks, who integrated it into a scientific system that would become the forerunner of our own. Aristotle, Hippocrates, and Galen, considered the fathers of modern medicine, all acknowledged the role of imagery in healing.[4]

Aristotle believed the emotional system did not function in the absence of images. Without the aid of modern technology, he realized that mental images caused changes in bodily function and affected both the cause and cure of disease. European medicine, in fact, was largely holistic until the time of Descartes, an influential French physician/philosopher of the early 17th century.

In his treatise on dualism, Descartes stated that the mind has nothing to do with the body, and the body has nothing to do with the mind.[5] This declaration left the mind and the soul completely under the jurisdiction of the Church, leaving Descartes free to dissect human cadavers without fear of retribution from the Pope. Whether Descartes actually believed this or not is uncertain. But his influence changed the course of Western medicine, setting the stage for the purely mechanical view of the human body it has held for the last four hundred years.

Imagery didn't make its way back into the medical discussion until the work of the Simontons in the late 1960s. Dr. O. Carl Simonton, a radiation oncologist, and his wife, Stephanie, a psychologist, demonstrated unexpected longevity in cancer patients who used visualization directed at boosting their immune systems.[6]

The Simontons' work sparked renewed interest in medical imagery and there has been much research on the subject in recent decades. Imagery has been shown to be useful in a wide range of conditions, including asthma, allergic reactions, pain management, high blood pressure, depression, and others. It has been used to speed healing after injuries as severe as broken bones, and to improve cancer patients' response to chemotherapy. There is virtually no disease process where imagery has not been shown to be helpful. Naparstek wonders why people don't use it every day, like aspirin.

Despite overwhelming evidence that healing imagery is beneficial, it remains on the fringes of Western medicine. Modern physicians consider themselves scientists much more than was the case fifty years ago, when house calls, a good bedside manner, and chicken soup were more in vogue. And imagery, by its very nature, smacks of being unscientific.

The gold standard of today's medicine is the randomized controlled trial (RCT). In an RCT, patients are randomly put into a group that receives some type of therapy or a control group that does not. The most rigorous RCTs are double-blinded and placebo-controlled, meaning the control group gets a placebo, but neither the patient nor the researcher knows who got the real medicine until all the data are collected.

The Power of Imagination

Unfortunately, imagery doesn't lend itself well to this type of analysis. We've already seen how difficult imagery is to define and how the different types overlap each other. What some call imagery, others call meditation, and still others would call prayer. And they *all* might be right.

It's not that RCTs don't show a benefit to imagery. They do—consistently. The problem is that imagery is harder for the medical mind to wrap itself around than CAT scans and laser surgery. Yes, there's a benefit, but is it imagery, or meditation, or something else altogether that's responsible for the benefit? It's impossible to distill things down to a single answer because it's all interconnected. This doesn't bother our intuitive side, but it drives our logical side crazy.

An RCT is a tool of the left brain, which is our logical, analytical, intellectual side. But imagery comes from the right brain, which is our creative, intuitive, artistic side. Using the strict criteria of an RCT to judge the value of imagery is like using a construction worker's toolbox to analyze a cloud. Hammers, wrenches, and screwdrivers are simply never going to do the job. Randomized controlled trials are wonderful research tools, but they're not the final word on reality.

Imagery, perhaps more than anything else, showcases the mind-body connection. Intangible thoughts govern hormone levels, blood pressure, and a host of very tangible things that can be measured easily in the lab. The Lemon Imagery proves that without even going to the lab. Your local movie theater proves the same thing. If you've ever gone to the movies and laughed or cried, or been angry or afraid, you've experienced imagery's power to effect physiologic change. They're just pictures. No one's actually up there on the screen.

For good or ill, imagery has the power to affect our health. And it's well documented. The fact that imagery isn't considered mainstream by modern medicine is more an indictment of modern medicine than a statement on the value of imagery.

How Does Imagery Work?

Part of the healing power of imagery has to do with its relaxing effects. Anything we do to counteract the chronic sympathetic overload so common to Western culture will have a positive effect on our health. But there's clearly more to it than that. Imagining immune cells performing highly specific functions and having them actually do it involves more than mere relaxation.

Naparstek calls sensory images "the true language of the body, the only language it understands immediately and without question." Studies show that imagery activates cortical areas of the brain in a similar way to actual events, which explains why our bodies can't differentiate between sensory images and what we call reality.[7]

This all makes sense within the same body: images that appear in *my* mind have an effect on *my* body. But what about the effects imagery has on events outside the body? It's one thing for mental rehearsal to improve one's performance in an individual game like golf, but what about sporting events involving players on other teams? And why do salesmen consistently perform better after spending time visualizing increased sales? It isn't all about them. Somebody else actually has to buy their wares.

This is not just a theoretical question. Remember, cancer is not something that just happens to us. It has to do with how we interact with the environment—and our mental images represent a major way we interact with the environment.

The images we carry in our heads—whether an echo of the past, a fear of the future, or self-created in the present—affect our physiology. But these same mental images also seem to affect the outside world. Yes, imagery is important to our health, but it may be more

The Power of Imagination

important to our life.

Modern science offers some explanations for how imagery works, and they have to do with our interconnectedness. We've already seen how freely interchangeable our atoms are. On an atomic level, there's no difference between my body and yours, or between us and the birds and the trees. The building blocks are completely interchangeable. Quantum physics tells us that the exchange of our energies is even more dynamic.

Quantum theory holds that everything in the universe is an interconnected mass of vibrating energy—including us. Objects differ only in the frequency of their vibration, with objects of lower frequencies perceived differently by our human senses than those of higher frequencies. In other words, everything in the universe is made of the same stuff. This resolves the quandary over how imagery can have an effect outside the body, because on one level of reality there is no outside.

The power of our intentions to affect the "outside" world is sometimes called The Law of Attraction. It states that one's vibrational frequency, which varies with the type of images we habitually hold in our minds, attracts people and objects of a similar frequency. Many consider the Law of Attraction controversial, but it not only agrees with what spiritual teachers have been telling us for millennia, it is a quantum physical reality.

Even for those well-versed in physics, it all gets very *meta*physical. Where do the images come from in receptive imagery, for instance? No one really knows. Some say they arise from our subconscious. Some say we have tapped into the Zero Point Field.* Others say we are hearing the voice of God. Personally speaking, I'm not sure I know the difference.

---

*The field of energy that underlies the universe. It exists everywhere at once, is connected to everything, and contains all knowledge of past, present, and future events.

Chapter Nine

Working with Imagery

Luckily, imagery is a lot easier to do than it is to explain. No one really understands how it works, but we don't have to know how it works to use it any more than we have to know how our car works to get in and drive.

As we touched on at the beginning of the chapter, working with imagery involves two steps. The first is simply learning to become aware of what's playing in the movie theater of our minds on a day-to-day basis. The resentments, worries, regrets—and judgments—of everyday life wreak havoc on our physiology if we don't keep them in check. The second step involves using mental movies we specifically create to help us overcome a life problem or a particular health issue.

Most of the interest in imagery has focused on the second type. It's much more glamorous to imagine your immune cells as soldiers destroying enemy cancer cells than it is to imagine yourself floating peacefully on a river with your worries standing by helplessly on the riverbank, unable to reach you. But this type of simple relaxation imagery is every bit as powerful as the more focused type. I would urge you not to leave it out.

Learning to avoid or counteract the stress-inducing negative imagery of worries, resentments, and petty irritations is powerful medicine. With practice, you can become aware of negative images as they start to creep in, and shift your focus to more positive images. This will improve not only your emotional health, but your physical health too.

For developing an imagery practice focused on a specific disease process, it's best to begin with guided imagery. *Guided Imagery for Self-healing* by Martin Rossman, M.D. is a good resource. Naparstek's *Staying Well With Guided Imagery* is excellent as well.

The Power of Imagination

Consider starting with a CD. The soothing voice of your guide, along with the background music, is helpful in inducing the relaxed state where imagery flows best. Reading the imageries in a book doesn't give you the same depth of experience, especially if you're a beginner. Naparstek's CDs are some of the best. She has recorded imageries designed specifically for cancer patients, and on many other subjects as well.

Developing an imagination practice is no different than acquiring any other habit. It takes time and perseverance. You may notice subtle changes in your life right away, but more obvious changes may take weeks or months. It isn't a quick fix, but if your goal is clear and you stick with it, your efforts will be richly rewarded. Above all, have fun with it. Like everything else in life, imagery comes easier when you don't take yourself so seriously.

I participated in an exercise called Wise Guide Imagery some years ago as part of a Center for Mind-Body Medicine (CMBM) small group. Imagery seemed strange to me in those days, but I was determined to keep an open mind. We were instructed to travel in our mind's eye along a path that passed by a field, meandered through the woods, and then led up to a clearing. There we would meet with whomever or whatever showed up in our imagination, and we could ask them anything we wished.

Not understanding at the time that the more vivid the images, the better the imagery, I found myself becoming impatient as our instructor "wasted time" prompting us to notice details about the field, what kind of shoes we were wearing, what the weather was like, and so on. I wanted to get to the clearing and get on with it, since I thought that was the point of the whole thing.

In my mind, I went right to the clearing, but the instructor's voice kept distracting me with comments meant to get me to focus on the path. It was uncomfortable trying to be in two places at once, so I reluctantly left the clearing and joined everyone else on the path. I again arrived at the clearing, this time presumably along with the rest of the group.

My wise guide that day was a large wolf and I'll never forget our "conversation." Still skeptical of the process, I thought I'd put it to the test. "What's the meaning of life?" I asked smugly. "Let's see what he does with *that*," I thought to myself. I wasn't going to throw out a cream puff question. I wanted to see if there was anything to this.

"If you keep rushing through life, always in a hurry to get to the next thing, you'll miss out on life entirely and you won't have to worry about the meaning of it," was the wolf's reply, delivered so fast it made my head spin.

It was as if my question had been anticipated and the answer made ready before I asked. No one could have possibly had time to think about it beforehand. I had to stifle my laughter so as not to disturb the rest of the group. The joke was obviously on me. Once it sunk in how profound the answer was, I was convinced.

Who was my wise guide that day? Who knows? The wolf was just a metaphor. The actual source is a matter of debate, and largely depends on your point of view. It's fine to debate the Who or the What—just don't miss the conversation.

An Exercise*

I'd like to bring this chapter to a close the same way we began, with an exercise. One that has the power to change your life if you're willing to spend some time with it. It's more of an assignment than an exercise, so feel free to read through the instructions a few times before you begin.

*Adapted from Deepak Chopra's *The Spontaneous Fulfillment of Desire*

The Power of Imagination

Start by finding a time and place where you won't be interrupted for twenty or thirty minutes, and sit down with a pen and a piece of paper. Breathe and relax for a minute or two, then begin the exercise by making a list of twenty things you want in life. That's it. Just make the list. Sounds easy enough, but like most things, there's more to it than meets the eye.

Coming up with twenty things may not be as easy as it sounds. Some of you may have trouble coming up with five or six, while others may quickly come up with sixty. If you're stuck at five, you may have never given serious thought to what's important to you. Keep working at it until you get twenty. If you come up with thirty or forty without any trouble, you may not be focused enough in your desires. Pare it down to twenty.

Don't write what you think you *should* want; write what you *really* want. Don't ask for world peace unless you're practicing for the Miss America pageant. Make it practical. This is for your eyes only, so don't hold back. If you want a better relationship with your spouse or your kids, write it down. If preventing breast cancer is a major concern, or losing weight, or any issue at all, put it down.

If you want material things, write them down, but consider using at least part of your "wishes" on self-image issues. Specific material needs are all well and good, but when your self-image changes—everything changes. Our self-image holds us back more than we know, and any move in a positive direction multiplies itself as it filters into every area of life. Self-image issues can also hold the key to our physical maladies in ways that are difficult to understand.

Write things down in the order they come to you. Don't judge what comes. Just write it down. There's a reason things come in the order they do. My spiritual life is very important to me, but when I first did this exercise, nothing even remotely spiritual came to me until number six. I was tempted to change it around so some of the more "selfish" things came closer to the bottom, but I thought better of it. There's something about being honest with yourself that adds power to the process.

When you get to twenty, begin to prioritize. If you think of something important that isn't on the list, add it by replacing something else. This is not a one-time exercise; it's an ongoing process. It may take several sittings to get your list to where you want it. There's no hurry; this is a meditation. Enjoy it.

Once you come up with twenty things, it's time to go back and adjust your list. Now's the time to change the order if you think some things should be given a higher priority. It's also important to be specific. Financial security, for instance, is too vague. Being able to pay all your bills at the end of the month would be a better place to start. Being healthy is too vague. Being off all your medications or being able to run three miles is more specific.

Make sure everything you listed is within the realm of believability for you. It should be enough of a stretch to excite you, but not so much of a stretch you consider it impossible. If your goal is to lose ten pounds over the next year, you could do that without any special imagery. If your goal is to lose fifty pounds in the next two weeks, you'll get discouraged quickly.

It's also important that your goals are stated in the positive. There's something about the way our minds are constructed that doesn't recognize the negative. If I asked you *not* to think of an elephant, for instance, you'd get a mental picture of an elephant. It takes a positive picture of a gorilla or a giraffe to make you forget about the elephant.

Goals such as not being in debt, not getting cancer, or not being judgmental, are counterproductive. They just get you focusing on debt, cancer, and being judgmental. And don't make it about losing a specific amount of weight. The "losing" is a negative; it just keeps you focused on your weight.

For most of us, thinking in the negative is deeply embedded in our psyche. It would be unusual if your list didn't need some work in this area. Change the wording around using only positive statements. This is about what you want; not what you don't want. This is very important.

Your list should be a good mix of short-term and long-term goals. If everything on your list isn't likely to happen for years, you won't stick with this practice long. Better to have too many short-term goals. As you achieve success with each goal, you'll gain confidence in the process. It's great positive feedback to cross an accomplished goal off the list and replace it with something else. Once you're satisfied that your list is a good mix of long and short-term goals, and is specific, believable, positive, and honest, you're ready to move on.

Now comes the fun part: simply take fifteen minutes every day and put your imagination to work on your list. You can spend more time if you like, but consistency is more important than the amount of time spent in any one sitting.

This is end-state imagery, so it's important to see whatever you're focusing on as a present reality. Don't imagine that it *will* happen. Imagine that it is happening or already has happened. When it seems so real that you feel a sense of gratitude for it, you know your imagery is having an effect.

It's important to be aware of your feelings during this process. They are the best barometer of its effectiveness. If you aren't feeling anything—nothing's happening. If the images don't at least make you smile, you're practicing what Naparstek calls two-dimensional imagery. This will not be as effective.

If you don't feel anything, it's a sign that your subconscious doesn't believe what your imagination is telling it. This is what happens with simple affirmations. You can say " I weigh 120 pounds" to yourself all day long, but if deep down you know you weigh 200, you might as well be talking to the wall.

An easy way around this internal resistance is to remind yourself that you're only *imagining* you weigh 120 pounds. You're not saying you actually do. If you want to be more confident, imagine for fifteen minutes a day that you *are* more confident. You don't struggle or pretend to be that way the rest of the day. Feel deeply what it would be like while you're practicing and then go about your normal life. There's no pressure in that. Add this small but important piece, and your subconscious will drop its resistance. Another way to accomplish the same thing is to ask yourself, "How would I feel if this goal were a present reality?" Then spend time reveling in the feeling.

Trust me, this is fun. When you can take fifteen minutes a day and imagine an ongoing problem into oblivion, it gets to be something you look forward to. After a time, you may find the process worthwhile in and of itself, regardless of whether the problem ever gets solved.

Is this an escape? Of course it is. But so is TV, shopping, gossiping about your neighbor, and a thousand other things. This, at least, has a positive purpose. Besides, you're only "escaping" from an external reality to an inner one. When you do this consistently, external reality changes.

None of this is to say that everything on your list is going to happen. It's also not to say that we can control external reality by mind power. We can't. It is to say that our intentions have more influence on our circumstances than we realize. Too few take advantage of it.

Breast Cancer and Your Imagination Practice

Your List of Twenty makes things simple in terms of breast cancer prevention. All you have to do is include a healthy diet, ideal body weight, stress reduction, and physical exercise goals on your list. And don't forget to reassess after you've finished the book, adding other risk-reducing practices we haven't discussed yet.

If you're at high risk for developing breast cancer, or you're a survivor seeking to prevent a recurrence, include a focused imagery specifically for prevention on your list. Be careful of the negativity aspect though. You may have to include breast cancer in your mental picture for it to be meaningful, but keep it in the periphery. Remember, you don't want to focus on what you don't want.

You might visualize yourself as being one of the Israelites during the first Passover in Egypt when they put lamb's blood on their doorposts to protect themselves from the spirit of death (in this case, breast cancer). If this fits with your religious tradition, it's a good one to go with. Images that have a deep spiritual meaning are some of the most powerful.

If you prefer something non-religious, you might see your immune system as a strong Coast Guard defending your coastline from invasion, or imagine your immune cells as Homeland Security agents, picking up terrorist cancer cells before they can take hold.

If you've been recently diagnosed with breast cancer, or are currently undergoing treatment, make sure to include a focused imagery based on healing your cancer. It might be a rocket ship type of imagery like Glen used, or it might be a type of cellular imagery focused on getting rid of the cancer cells. As always, the best imagery is the one that's the most meaningful to you.

Chapter Nine

Key Points to Remember

- Be specific.
- State your goals in the positive.
- Include self-image issues.
- Be honest.
- Make it believable.
- Bypass internal resistance.
- If you're smiling, it's going great.
- Have fun.

If you decide to embark on an imagination practice, you will be in good company. World-class athletes have used visualization techniques for years. Thomas Edison was well known for using imagery. This makes perfect sense, since an invention is something that does not currently exist. Who could invent anything without first "seeing" it in their mind's eye?

Perhaps the most famous person to make extensive use of imagination was Albert Einstein. Despite what many think, Einstein was not a good student. Because he couldn't find an academic position after graduate school, he took a job as a clerk at the patent office in Bern, Switzerland.

In 1905, while working at the patent office, he published three papers that catapulted him to fame, including his Theory of Relativity. His experiments were largely imagination experiments, many based on his musings about the trains he saw pulling in and out of the station across the street.

If Einstein could do what he did while working as a patent office clerk, there's no telling what's possible for you. To those who know how to use their imagination, the improbable is commonplace. Einstein had this to say about it:

The Power of Imagination

"Imagination is more important than knowledge, for
knowledge is limited to all we know and understand, while
imagination embraces the entire world, and all there
ever will be to know and understand....Logic will get you
from A to B. Imagination will get you everywhere."

ༀ

10
Understanding Your Emotions

৵

Breast cancer is an emotional subject. It evokes strong feelings—even in women who are never diagnosed with it. Understanding your emotions and being able to manage them effectively is a crucial skill, not only in the breast cancer process, but also in life. It gives you a degree of control no matter what's happening around you.

Unfortunately, most of us are emotionally illiterate. We don't know what emotions are. We don't know what they're for. And we don't know what to do with them when they show up. Because of this, most of us experience our emotions passively. They run us instead of us running them.

Emotions are as powerful as they are mysterious. Because they sometimes make us feel out of control, we tend to avoid them and focus on our intellectual side. But feelings are fundamental to our experience of life. As we've just seen with imagery, our emotions are an accurate measure of what's happening within us on a deeper level. Shutting them down because they're uncomfortable may work in the short run, but in the long run it's not an effective strategy.

Chapter Ten

Emotions and Cancer

Chronically repressing emotions is felt by many to be an actual risk factor for breast cancer. This is well accepted in Traditional Chinese Medicine (TCM), where repression of emotions is considered to be a risk factor for cancer in general. Even in the West, some experts have long suspected this to be true. In the second century A.D., Galen noted that cancer was much more frequent in "melancholic" than "sanguine" women.[1]

James Paget (1870), in his textbook, *Surgical Pathology,* stated that "The cases are so frequent in which deep anxiety, deferred hope and disappointment are quickly followed by the growth and increase of cancer, we can hardly doubt that mental depression is a weighty addition to the other influences favoring the development of a cancerous constitution."[2]

An 1893 study from the London Cancer Hospital, one of the first statistical analyses of the effects of psychological factors on the development of cancer, concluded that "The number of instances in which malignant disease of the breast and uterus follows immediately antecedent emotion of a depressing character is too large to be set down to chance."[3]

The results of more recent statistical analyses have been mixed, some showing a correlation between emotions and breast cancer incidence, and some not. In those that do, chronic repression of anger is a recurring theme.[4] In breast cancer patients the findings are less controversial. Women who show the ability to express their emotions live longer and have a better quality of life than those who don't.[5]

Studies may not consistently show a direct link between emotions and cancer risk, but indirect evidence is abundant and convincing. A significant portion of the obesity problem, for instance, is due to eating out of *emotional* hunger rather than physical hunger. The term "comfort food" speaks to this reality. Food wasn't meant to comfort us, it was meant to meet our nutritional needs.

Depression can also cause us to overeat. Food gives us an immediate boost in energy, but it is not designed to be a sustained mood-enhancer. Those who use food in this manner tend to consume a lot of it. People who are depressed also tend to exercise less, making depression a double threat to breast cancer risk.

From a holistic perspective, it seems obvious that emotions have a strong effect on breast cancer risk. The effect is overlooked in research studies because it is one step removed from more easily measurable parameters such as diet and exercise. But the effect is there, and the message is clear—address the underlying emotional issues, and the overeating goes away. Regardless of the breast cancer question, so-called toxic emotions are well known to damage our health.

According to Daniel Goleman, author of *Emotional Intelligence*, "Helping people better manage their upsetting feelings—anger, anxiety, depression, pessimism, and loneliness—is a form of disease prevention." The toxicity of these emotions, when chronic, is on a par with smoking cigarettes. Helping people handle them better could potentially have a medical payoff as great as getting heavy smokers to quit.[6]

Emotional Intelligence

Most of us are on emotional autopilot. We react emotionally the same way our parents did, not because they told us we should, but because no one ever talked about it. Children don't so much learn their parents' emotional patterns as they absorb them.

Luckily, we are no more tied to our emotional patterns by

Chapter Ten

heredity than we are to cancer risk. We inherit emotional tendencies, but these are not fixed. Like breast cancer risk, they can be modified.

Knowing that you can modify your emotional patterns is empowering. It gives you a degree of control in yet another area where you likely thought you had none. It may decrease your risk of breast cancer, but it will certainly improve your experience of life. Your emotions are a pathway to understanding yourself; a window into your soul—a guide to a better life.

According to Daniel Goleman, 80% of adult success is based on "emotional intelligence (EQ)," which he defines as having an "awareness of our emotions and the ability to manage them in a healthy and productive manner." Your EQ is a far more reliable predictor of success *in any endeavor* than how smart you are (IQ). Enhancing your emotional intelligence will allow you to negotiate any crisis more effectively—or avoid one altogether.

Emotional Awareness

It is impossible to do any work with our emotions unless we are aware of what we're feeling. There is a general lack of awareness concerning our feelings in Western culture, which can be seen in the words we use to describe them. When asked how we feel, we often respond with words like "rejected," "insulted," or "humiliated." But these aren't truly feelings—they're thoughts and opinions.

The words themselves tell a story, but the story is incomplete. Another actor is required for the scene to make any sense. In order to be rejected, I have to be rejected *by* someone. The same is true with being humiliated or insulted. These are basically my stories about what someone "did to me." They are my interpretation of events—a story that may or may not be true. In terms of stressful emotions, facts are nothing. The story we tell ourselves about the facts is everything.

There is an eye-opening discussion about this in Dr. Marshall Rosenberg's book, *Nonviolent Communication*. Rosenberg emphasizes that **emotional awareness begins with making the distinction between what we feel and what we think.**

The following is a partial list of words commonly used to describe our emotions. The words on the left reflect our opinions, interpretations, or stories, even though we often use these words to describe our feelings. The words in the center are actual feelings we would describe as pleasant, and on the right, feelings we consider less pleasant. A more complete list can be found in Dr. Rosenberg's book:[7]

abandoned	affectionate	angry
betrayed	appreciative	annoyed
bullied	cheerful	apathetic
coerced	confident	ashamed
intimidated	delighted	brokenhearted
let down	energetic	confused
manipulated	encouraged	dejected
neglected	happy	depressed
overworked	hopeful	disappointed
patronized	joyful	embarrassed
pressured	mellow	fearful
put down	optimistic	frustrated
rejected	peaceful	gloomy
taken for granted	proud	lethargic
threatened	relaxed	lonely
unappreciated	secure	nervous
unheard	trusting	resentful

Chapter Ten

If you're like most of us, you've found yourself using words from the left column to describe how you feel—even though they're not feelings. If you want to try a lighthearted exercise with your partner, sit down sometime and talk about how you feel without using any of the "illegal" words from the column on the left. It's more difficult than you might think, and can be quite amusing. When it comes to how we feel, we don't say what we mean, not because we're dishonest, but because we simply don't have the vocabulary.

Once we've identified what we feel, **it's important to acknowledge the feeling as our own.** Our emotions are *our* emotions. Outside circumstances may trigger them, but they do not technically cause them. No one "makes" us mad, or "makes" us sad. We can only do that ourselves. Others may pull the trigger on our emotions, but it's our gun and it only exists in our head. Sometimes others' behavior is abominable, true enough, but making them responsible for what we feel is a path to nowhere.

When we use words like "rejected," "unappreciated," or "abandoned" to describe how we feel, we are doing much the same with our emotions as we so often do with our stress—blame someone else for it. Blaming something outside of ourselves for how we feel is comforting, but it's disempowering. We escape responsibility for our feelings, at least in our own minds, but our personal power escapes along with it because we've just given it away to the one we've blamed.

Reclaiming responsibility for our emotions can be disconcerting at first, but we can't make any headway in managing our emotions as long as we disown them. When we own what we feel, it empowers us—even if we don't like what we're feeling. Taking responsibility for our emotions is a major step in taking control of our lives.

It is also helpful to **identify where in the body you feel an emotion**. Emotions can usually be perceived in a specific location in the body. Many emotions are perceived in the chest area, but they can be felt anywhere. The old sayings, "a pain in the neck," and "getting it off our chest," are more than just metaphors.

Being able to localize an emotion to a particular area in your body shows increasing self-awareness. The feeling is there. Whether you're aware of it or not is the only question. As with anything else, becoming aware is largely a matter of paying attention and practice.

Most of us would like to feel all the things from the center column of Rosenberg's list, while feeling none of the things on the right. Unfortunately, that's not how things work. To the degree you shut down any emotion, you shut down all emotions. Our unwillingness to feel our fear, anger, or sadness automatically results in a diminished capacity to feel joy, gratitude, and love.

Avoiding fear and suppressing anger takes a bigger toll than just a physical one. It diminishes our experience of life. Our emotions give color and texture to our lives. Without them, life has little meaning.

Once we're aware of what we're feeling, where we're feeling it, and have taken full responsibility for it, we have to decide what we're going to do with it. It's here. It's ours. Now what?

Is it Really an Emergency?

Knowing what to do next is easier when we understand the nature and purpose of emotions. The word emotion is derived from the Latin roots, *ex-*, meaning "out of," and *movere*, meaning "to move." Quite literally, our emotions are a means of getting us to "move out," or to take action of some kind. Every emotion has something it's trying to tell us. Sometimes the message has to do with others. Sometimes it has to do with us. The trick is knowing how and when to listen so we can tell the difference.

Chapter Ten

Understanding the physiology of stress helps us know how and when to listen. Remember, there are many different types of stress but only one physiologic response. When we're experiencing emotional stress, we're in survival mode. Blood flow is shunted away from the brain and into the muscles. We're ready to fight or run away, but we're not equipped to make rational decisions.

Modern culture is a relatively recent invention. Our survival responses are wired for a different world altogether than the one most of us live in. It's critical to remember this when our survival mechanisms are triggered. Our physical eyes may be seeing our spouse, our boss, or rush hour traffic, but our physiology is seeing saber-tooth tigers, bears, and herds of stampeding mammoths.

When we are emotionally stressed, it's always a good idea to cool down and make sure our eyes and our physiology are seeing the same thing before making any decisions. If we act immediately out of strong negative emotion, we will be listening to a message from the primordial jungle and applying it to modern society—often with disastrous results.

It is emotionally intelligent to wait until we're in a mental state conducive to making rational decisions before making any. You don't want to make a social or relational decision while you're in survival mode. You only want to make survival decisions in survival mode.

Sometimes anger is immediately protective. Sometimes we really do need to defend ourselves—right now. So, take action right now if you need to. Otherwise, it's a good idea to let your physiology return from its brief trip to the jungle so you can get a more modern translation of the message.

Aristotle said, "Anyone can become angry—that is easy. But to be angry with the right person, to the right degree, at the right time, for the right purpose, and in the right way—that is not easy." This is impossible to do if we react immediately out of strong emotion. It's always good to *be* in the moment. It's not always good to *act* in the moment.

Move the Energy On

The physiology of the stress response makes one thing clear: you will *not* make good decisions under the influence of strong negative emotion because the emotion itself distorts the message. Except for a true emergency, rare in the modern world, the wisest thing to do is move the emotional energy on, then reconsider the situation.

How do we move it on? Breathe, first of all. Take a few deep cleansing breaths and then go into the "deeper, slower, quieter, more rhythmic" pattern. This will take the edge off quickly. Then move. Emotional stress is just stress, and emotional energy is just energy. Use it up any way that suits you. Shake. Dance. Exercise. Whatever your favorite form of movement—just do it.

Simply giving voice to you're experience is also an effective way to move emotional energy on. Tell a close friend or a counselor what's going on with you. It doesn't matter who. What matters is that you get it off your chest. Don't dump the emotion on them; just tell them about it. This isn't about venting your anger or indulging your fears. It's about giving voice to them.

This is an incredibly valuable process. Some have suggested the increased survival in Dr. Spiegel's patients was more due to the group setting that allowed women to express their emotions rather than the imagery. Just having someone you can talk to honestly, without being judged for it, is tremendously healing.

If there's no one to talk to, you can accomplish the same thing in a journal. The value of journaling as a way of expressing emotions is well documented.[8,9] A beautiful example comes from the diary of

Chapter Ten

Pat Tillman, as quoted in Jon Krakauer's recent book, *Where Men Win Glory: The Pat Tillman Story*.[10]

Tillman, an all-pro safety with the Arizona Cardinals of the NFL, turned down a multi-million dollar contract offer from the Cardinals in 2002 to join the Army Rangers and go fight in Afghanistan. In April 2004, he was killed in a friendly fire incident in Khost Province, near the Pakistani border. Because of his status as a former NFL player and the tragic circumstances of his death, his loss was felt by the nation.

Near the end of boot camp, prior to being deployed, Tillman felt frustrated and disillusioned. Having second thoughts and missing his beloved wife, Marie, he wrote:

> Sometimes I feel an injection of intense sorrow that is difficult to control, an intense need to be close to Marie, grounded by her touch, smell, sound, beauty and ease. It's as though one week of pain is condensed into five to seven minutes. What have I done?

> ...In a way it is refreshing in that this place has yet to callous or numb me. Somehow I enjoyed letting myself long for my wife and the life I left behind. It makes me feel and appreciate, and love. It makes me feel very alive and aware of my struggle...life is about feeling and emotion. Love, laughter and joy, as well as pain, longing and sorrow are all part of the ride. Without the latter, you cannot truly appreciate the former....

> I am experiencing and growing, and with this comes some suffering, but it's part of the deal....Passion is what makes life interesting...[It] ignites our soul, drives our curiosity, fuels our love and carries our friendships....A passion for life is contagious, and uplifting. Passion cuts both ways. Those [emotions] that make you feel on top of the world are equally able to turn it upside down....

> I want to create passion in my own life and with those I care for. I want to feel, experience and live every emotion. I will suffer through the bad for the heights of the good....

Understanding Your Emotions

Tillman's sensitivity and emotional maturity are surprising for someone so young. It's not what you'd expect from a stereotypical NFL player and Army Ranger. It has been said that at the end of our lives we will only have to answer two questions: "Did I live fully?" and "Did I love well?" Tillman obviously did both.

It takes courage to face difficult emotions, but if we don't, we miss much of life's beauty. Feeling a wide range of emotions is healthy. Exhibiting a limited range of emotions or holding on to the same emotion for long periods of time, are signs that something is amiss. Emotions change like the weather. They're meant to. The world we live in is constantly changing. If our emotions don't reflect that fact, we may not be relating to it in an appropriate way.

Feelings are meant to be felt, acted on appropriately, and moved on. When we short-circuit this natural flow, we set the stage for illness. Like any form of energy, emotional energy doesn't just dissipate on its own. Unless we make use of it, it's stored in our bodies. If you apply energy to any object in the known universe consistently over time, without allowing the object to discharge the energy, the object will eventually either break down or explode. The human body is no different.

Emotional energy that isn't moved on becomes "stuck," which can create serious health problems. If we don't keep the flow going, sadness becomes depression, fear leads to paranoia, anger becomes hostility, and anxiety turns into panic. Even positive emotions can become stuck. It isn't appropriate to feel cheerful, energetic, and confident all the time.

Women tend to repress anger perhaps more than any other emotion. When anger comes to their door, they don't shoot the messenger so much as tie him up, gag him, and lock him in the basement. After years of the same emotional pattern, it gets crowded down there—and toxic. And it's more than just a metaphor. Chronic repressed anger is a stronger predictor of dying young—from any cause—than smoking, high blood pressure, and high cholesterol.[11]

Our emotions are like the tides—they come and go, and come again. When we resist this natural flow, we pay a high price, mentally, spiritually, *and* physically. It's important to allow them to come, but just as important to let them go.

Listen for the Deeper Message

Once we've ruled out an emergency and moved the emotional energy on, we're ready to get to the heart of the issue, which is listening to the deeper message. Don't rush into this, but don't let too much time pass, either. When it's appropriate, spend some time searching out your feelings. They carry a wealth of information. Just remember, the message is just as often about your own attitude as it is someone else's conduct. Even if someone is being a "bad actor," our emotional stress is more about us than it is about them.

Every emotion carries a different message. Even the message from the same emotion can be different at different times. Still, there are overriding themes. Sadness and grief, for instance, are usually telling us it's time to slow down. If we have recently lost a loved one, it takes time for our bodies to readjust to life without them. After a loss, emotional healing is just as necessary as it is with a physical wound. Grief slows us down for a reason. We don't feel like doing anything because we don't *need* to be doing anything. Our bodies need the time to heal. Our feelings of sadness encourage us to take the time.

Anger usually has to do with protection. It tells us someone has violated our rights. If we never stand up for ourselves, anger continues to build. Our anger may be telling us we need to set a boundary of some sort. When we set the boundary, the anger subsides because it has done its job. If we don't, the anger will become a recurring theme because we haven't heeded the message.

It isn't always that simple, of course. Emotions are a complex web, with deeper layers and subtle nuances. Anger often masks a deeper loneliness, hurt, or fear. This is typical in men, many of whom were raised with the subtle or not-so-subtle message that it isn't okay to cry, but it's okay to be angry. Crying usually comes easier for women because most were raised with the message that it's okay to cry, but not to be angry.

These are cultural generalities, of course. Each of us is emotionally unique. The point is, when an emotion shows up we need to pay close attention to it. There will always be something it asks of us, whether it's taking steps to protect ourselves or looking deeper into our own hearts.

When a course of action isn't obvious, it's time to go deeper. Getting in touch with our inner wisdom or our higher power can give us the answer we're looking for—if we take the time to listen.

To Sum Up

The healthiest way to deal with any emotion is to **feel it, name it, and own it.** Know what you're feeling and where in the body you feel it. Remember the difference between what you feel and what you think. **If you need to protect yourself—act. If not—wait.** Emotional intelligence is as much about what you don't do as what you do. Waiting out a strong emotion without taking action is the most difficult part of the process, but it's the clearest sign you are maturing in it.

Not taking immediate action on strong emotion isn't stuffing it. It shows you know the difference between the modern world and the ancient one. Promising yourself you will take appropriate action at the proper time will in itself lessen the intensity of the emotion.

Move the emotional energy on. Once you've agreed to hear the message at a more appropriate time, the emotion has done its job—it has alerted you. It doesn't benefit you to wallow in it. Breathe. Move. Talk to a friend. Journal. Move some more. Do whatever it takes to dissipate the energy. When you're feeling more like yourself, you'll have a better perspective on the event that triggered your emotion.

Once you've calmed down, you're ready to **listen to the deeper message,** which is basically a meditation on your emotions. If you're willing to get quiet and ask questions—the answers will come. And **once you've heard the message, don't forget to act on it**. Otherwise the whole process has been for naught.

Any emotion can be considered good if it is acknowledged, experienced fully, the energy moved on, and the message received and acted upon. No emotions are bad, not even the unpleasant ones. They all have something important to tell us, perhaps *especially* the unpleasant ones. Toxic emotions aren't toxic because they're uncomfortable; they're toxic only when we get stuck in them.

Having a deeper understanding of your emotions will be a major benefit in every area of life, breast cancer notwithstanding. The question, "What am I feeling right now?" is the beginning of emotional wisdom. Ask it often, even if you fumble with the answer. Ask it—and keep on asking it—and you will grow in self-awareness. Knowing what to do with your feelings will come in time. There's more value in the question than there is in having the perfect answer.

Knowing what we are feeling in the moment is a coming home of sorts. For many of us, it is getting reacquainted with ourselves. Looking into our own hearts and acknowledging, "I feel sad," "I am afraid," or "I feel lonely," is something most of us rarely do, perhaps because it requires us to come to terms with the frailest parts of ourselves. When we can meet those parts of ourselves—without

Understanding Your Emotions

blaming anyone for them—we open an inner door. When we can hold them with tenderness and compassion, we're home to stay. ❧

11

The Importance of
Healthy Relationships

❧

Nowhere does emotional intelligence pay higher dividends than in your relationships. And nothing pays higher dividends for your health than having good ones. We've already mentioned that wound healing can be delayed up to 24 hours after a marital argument.[1] Those who have troubled relationships have higher rates of disease and premature death.[2] In other words, your immune system is less effective when you are in conflict with your spouse or companion.

Having close emotional support is critical for your health, the occasional marital disagreement notwithstanding. Not only is the incidence of cancer lower among married people, but cancer patients who are married survive longer than those who are single, separated, widowed, or divorced.[3]

It isn't just about marriage—it's about the quality of *all* your relationships. Many studies show higher rates of cancer in those who do not have a strong social network.[4] Cancer patients without such a network do not survive as long as those who do. In fact, the risk of death from *any* cause is two to five times higher in those who describe themselves as socially isolated as compared to those who are socially engaged.[5]

Simply put, the health of your relationships affects your physical health. In terms of reproducible scientific proof, it's a slam-dunk. According to Dean Ornish, M.D., author of *Love and Survival*, "Love and intimacy are among the most powerful factors in health and illness." Part of the reason Dr. Spiegel's breast cancer patients survived twice as long as their counterparts was almost certainly due to the quality relationships they forged in his group. The group met for only a year, but the relationships were lasting ones.

The link between relationships and health is another overlooked subject by the medical community, perhaps because a relationship isn't a physical entity. You can't X-ray it, treat it with medication, or perform surgery on it. And yet it affects your health dramatically.

Traditional medicine may overlook the impact of relationships on your health, but you shouldn't. It is a critical part of any self-care plan. Dr. Ornish lays out the simple choice we have when it comes to our intimate relationships:[6]

Commitment		Fear/no commitment
⇩		⇩
Trust		Mistrust
⇩	*or:*	⇩
Vulnerability		Hostility
⇩		⇩
Intimacy		Isolation
⇩		⇩
Healing		Disease/premature death

Relationships are often the first thing to be neglected in stressful times, but they shouldn't be because relational stress will only add to whatever stress you already have. Consistently putting your relationship on the back burner is never a good idea. When a crisis hits, if you've been doing routine maintenance on your relationship it will help keep you afloat. If you haven't it can drag you under. We mop the floor, we dust the shelves, we change the oil in the car, but somehow we expect our relationships to work by themselves. They don't.

A relationship can be compared to a bank account. If you always borrow and never deposit, you may find your relationship overdrawn when you need it most. Any time and effort you put into it is a good investment, both for your health and your overall enjoyment of life.

Don't wait until you feel like it or until your partner "deserves" it. Any kindness is more powerful when it's not particularly deserved. This touches on a larger discussion of grace. Suffice it to say here that relationships where grace is given and received freely are the most successful ones.

A Little Background

I'd like to share a little of my own story at this point, just so you'll know my relationship "credentials." Like most of us, I got the bulk of my relationship training in the school of hard knocks. It's a popular school. It's easy to get in, and tuition is free. The catch is, it takes a lot of hard work to get out. Most of us fall into it early in life out of ignorance and spend the rest of our lives looking for ways not to go back.

I have been married to the same woman for 30 years, more or less. No, I haven't forgotten my anniversary. There's a reason I can't tell you how long I've been married. But let's start at the beginning.

Lana and I met shortly before our 15th birthdays while attending the same high school in Southern Maryland. On the second day of school, I transferred into her Latin class where the only seat available was right in front of her. We hit it off immediately, quickly becoming friends. We began dating the following year and later attended the same college, marrying after our junior year, at age 20.

It seemed like a match made in heaven. The years went by, we had four wonderful children, and life was humming along nicely. Until from out of nowhere—the crisis hit. It wasn't from out of nowhere, of course; it just seemed that way because we weren't paying attention. There were plenty of warning signs, but we ignored them all.

After eleven years as an Army physician, I had just left the military for private practice, taking a new job in a new state, with too many hours, and too much turmoil. We were building our dream home at the same time, *and* adjusting to life with two adolescents, a toddler and a newborn.

It was an overwhelming amount to take on, but didn't seem so at the time. Sure it was difficult, but everything had always worked out and we were certain things would settle down eventually. We were on autopilot. Unfortunately, the road took a sharp turn—and the autopilot didn't.

We didn't know much about stress at the time, but it's clear now we were asking for trouble. Stress doesn't just kill the physical body. Relationships also die by its cruel hand. We made the mistake of thinking it could never happen to us—but it did.

Divorces are rarely quick and never simple. And ours was no exception. It was a drawn-out, painful affair that took several years to sort out. Families don't separate along neat perforated lines; they tear apart with jagged edges. Things may look clean and simple on the surface, but on the level of the soul, they're anything but.

We weathered it as well as anyone could, I suppose. I bought a place just ten minutes away and we spent holidays together, continuing our family traditions. On the surface we did pretty well.

The Importance of Healthy Relationships

Underneath we were both devastated.

Life normalized over time, though we had gotten together at such a young age it was hard to know what normal was. We were apart six years, more or less. I can't remember exactly when we signed the divorce papers.

We saw each other frequently because there were always ball games and graduations and recitals to attend. Things had become easier, and our friendship slowly returned. After a time, finding ourselves both unattached, we began to think about the unthinkable—getting back together.

We had both done a lot of personal work while we were apart. Lana had gotten a graduate degree in mental health counseling, and I had attended numerous relationship classes and seminars. We had always loved each other and it had been a while since the really hard times. Although neither of us thought it would be easy, we thought it worth the risk, especially with a family at stake.

I had planned a trip to Israel that summer, and we decided that both of us should go, along with children, and we'd have a ceremony over there. It was a wild idea, but we figured, why not? It took some arranging but we pulled it off, and were remarried during our tour of the Holy Land in the summer of 1999. Standing near the Mount of Olives overlooking the old city of Jerusalem, we made our vows—children by our side and two busloads of fellow-tourists as guests.

"This is a miracle," I remember saying to myself as I glanced around during the ceremony. Here I was, being reunited with my lifelong friend, in a setting that was nothing short of magical. Lana looked just as beautiful as she did at our first wedding. "How did this all this even happen?" I wondered. "How could such a nightmare turn into *this*?" Had I been given the script to write myself, I couldn't have written it so beautifully.

Our tour leader, an ordained minister, performed the ceremony,

Chapter Eleven

but had no credentials in Israel. When we returned home we wanted to make it legal, so we had a reception near our home in Naples, Florida for friends and family who weren't able to make the trip to Israel.

We decided to exchange vows again at the reception so everyone could share the occasion. It was a wonderful time, but in all the commotion of people coming and going, we neglected to sign the papers. So we *still* weren't legally married, even after another ceremony.

Two months later, on Lana's birthday, we met on the beach with our friend Gary, the minister who had performed the ceremony at our reception. We said a few more quick vows—we pretty much knew them by heart at this point—and finally signed the papers. Gary joked with us about the multiple ceremonies, saying God wanted to be sure it "took" this time.

So there you have it: an unusual story to say the least, and four anniversaries counting the original one. Which one do we celebrate? All of them. We feel like we've earned them, so why not? And if we happen to miss one, there's always another one right around the corner.

Now you understand why I can't tell you exactly how long we've been married. I honestly don't know. I could figure it out with some detective work, but I don't want to. It's more fun this way. When someone asks us how long we've been married, Lana and I look at each other with a smile and reply, "How much time do you have?"

How's it going? Well, it hasn't been that easy, but it hasn't been that hard either. It's been work, but part of the problem the first time was we didn't think it should be. It's taken time, effort, and some heartache—building anything of value always does. Nearly twelve years later, we both consider it a success. With each passing year it becomes harder to remember what all the commotion was about.

The Importance of Healthy Relationships

To recreate a family with the original pieces has been a blessing—perhaps my greatest blessing in a life that's been full of them. I know the odds of couples that remarry their former spouse staying together are abysmally low, but this book is all about defying the odds, isn't it?

In looking back at it all—what's gone right and what's gone wrong, what I wish I had known, and what I wish I had done—a few things stand out. There are a lot of relationship skills I wish I'd had earlier, but three I now consider indispensible: empathetic listening, understanding projection, and forgiveness.

Empathetic Listening

Learning to be a better listener is guaranteed to improve your relationship, no matter what its present state. No other skill is so simple, yet so profound in its positive effect on a relationship.

Most of us confuse hearing with actual listening, even though the two are quite different. Hearing requires only your ears, and a (surprisingly) few brain cells. Listening requires your whole being. You hear with your ears, but you listen with your soul. Effective listening is never casual. It requires you to be fully present. If you've ever said to a frustrated partner, "I *am* listening," you probably weren't.

This type of listening has been called empathetic listening to distinguish it from mere mechanical hearing. Empathy has been described as a respectful understanding of what others are experiencing. It is an emptying of the mind and listening with your whole being. It is an active process, not a passive one.

According to Daniel Goleman, 90 percent or more of human communication is nonverbal. If we are to really understand what our partners are feeling, we have to pay attention to the subtleties in their body language and voice inflections. It requires our full attention and some detective work, but the rewards are great if we're willing to make the effort.

A Few Listening Pointers

The bad news about empathetic listening is that few of us do it well. The good news is that anyone can learn to do it better. It's never too late to start.

Listening can be considered a meditation because it requires focus and attention. Meditative listening is fundamentally no different than focusing your attention on a single point or a mantra. Because your intention is to connect with another human soul, however, the potential rewards are higher.

Common listening mistakes have to do with not being fully present. Multitasking, for instance, is a communication killer. If you're trying to do something else and listen at the same time, you won't do either one well. Trust me, you'll pay a higher relationship price for not listening, so whatever else you're tempted to do at the same time, put it on hold.

Focusing on your own thoughts while your partner is speaking, or formulating a rebuttal while they're still talking, are signs of not being fully present. These are forms of mental multitasking. The tendency to finish others' sentences for them is a sure sign of this. Just because you're not talking while they are doesn't mean you're listening.

Empathetic listening requires you to temporarily put aside your needs and focus on those of your partner. An argument can be defined as two people trying to be heard without anyone actually listening. Until someone takes the first step, nothing's going to change. The difficulty, of course, is that our egos hate to listen. The ego wants its opinions heard. It doesn't want to take a back seat to anyone.

Remember that you're only *temporarily* putting your needs aside. This will help ease your pain. You'll get your turn to be heard. Assure your ego of that as you're putting it away while you listen to your partner. It will kick and scream a little less.

Don't be distracted by the words. Successful listening is not in hearing someone's words; it's in hearing their heart. Why should we focus all our attention on the words when they account for only a small percentage of what's really going on? Focusing only on the words is like pretending the visible part of an iceberg is all that exists. It was the invisible part of the iceberg that sank the Titanic, and it's the feelings beneath the words that sink relationships.

Listening is an active process, not a passive one. Listen with all your senses. Pay attention to your partner's body language and their facial expressions. Do they seem peaceful, nervous, excited, worried? What are they really asking for? Often it's only our undivided attention.

Effective listening is not complete silence. In fact, complete silence may be a sign of not being totally engaged. Ask for more detail. Paraphrase what you think you're hearing to make sure you have it right. Be interested. What they're saying may not be important to you, but it's important to them—and *they're* important to you. This is the message you send by giving your full attention. It is a message of caring and respect.

Don't judge. Just listen. Passing judgment on what's being said is another communication killer. When you judge, you're listening to your own self-righteousness, not to your partner. Good listening is being present with the speaker, regardless of what's being said. Appreciate that what they're saying is valid for them. It doesn't have to be valid for you. Put the Judge away wherever you put your ego.

It will make a mess of things if you don't.

Don't fix. Don't analyze. Just listen. Attempting to fix someone's problems, or worse yet trying to fix the person, is a definite no-no. Although often done with good intentions, fixing and analyzing are perceived as harsh acts. It's best to resist the urge. Besides, most of us don't need or want you to fix everything. We just want to be heard.

Being a good listener does not mean allowing yourself to be a garbage dump for gossip and complaints. If you find yourself in this situation, do the speaker a favor and change the subject, even if you have to interrupt. If they persist in the negativity, just walk away. You'll be doing both them and yourself a favor.

Communication is a team game. The two most common "speaker errors" are speaking under the influence of strong emotion and blaming your partner for what you feel. The two most common "listening errors" are not being fully present and being defensive.

The speaker sets the tone by how he or she speaks, but even if it's not done perfectly, the listener can make it work by refusing to take it personally. Whatever the speaker feels is about them, not you. As the listener, it pays to remember this—even if the speaker doesn't.

Expect to fail—often. Just don't quit trying. Listening is simple, but it isn't easy. Don't expect to get it right the first time, or the first ten times. Choose your topics wisely in the beginning. Practice talking about the toothpaste for a while before you tackle finances, sex, or the in-laws.

Empathetic, compassionate, non-defensive listening is one of the most healing things one human can do for another. Simply being present and listening from the heart sends a message of deep caring and compassion. This type of listening is a gift. Give it as often as you can.

Projection

Projection is a psychological defense mechanism where a person unconsciously denies his or her own attributes, thoughts, or emotions, which are then ascribed to other people. Freud originally coined the term, but the concept is much older than that.

In the New Testament, Jesus encourages us to *Be...perfect, even as your Father in Heaven is perfect* (Matthew 5:48 KJV). It's an unusual verse, one that on the surface would seem to have little to do with your relationship. We all know how detrimental trying to be perfect or requiring perfection of your partner is.

Things become clearer when we recall that the New Testament was originally written in Greek. The word "perfect" in this passage comes from the Greek word *teleios*, which can also be translated as "complete" in the sense of mental or moral completeness.

A universally accepted aspect of the divine is that it is completely integrated. It is everywhere at once, all knowing, and all powerful. There are many different aspects of God's character, but no aspect of God that is separate from the Whole; no part that isn't aware of every other part. It simply isn't possible.

As humans, we also have many aspects of our personality. In the state of mental disease this becomes evident as Multiple Personality Disorder. It's only logical, however, that there can't be a Multiple Personality *Dis*order unless there is a Multiple Personality *Order* to begin with. This is where the story of projection begins.

All of us are born fully integrated, meaning we're fully in touch with our various parts. Sometimes infants are irritable, sometimes they're happy. Sometimes they cry, sometimes they laugh. Sometimes they're blissfully content, and at other times quite demanding. The baby doesn't judge any of these states as far as we know. The baby just is. He or she accepts them as the way things are in the moment.

Chapter Eleven

As the child grows, however, things get more complicated. Some of these states are deemed unacceptable by authority figures. Imperfect parents rarely get the message across that it's the behavior that's unacceptable rather than the child. And so begins the unconscious process of shutting down these parts of the child's personality. Why *wouldn't* they shut them down if expressing them causes the child to be rejected?

The parts deemed unacceptable differ in every family. Some children are never allowed to show anger. Sometimes it isn't okay to express any emotion at all. As children, we learn to please the adults around us. We will get love any way we can because it's what we need the most. If shutting down parts of ourselves is the price of love, we'll gladly pay it.

Each facet of our personality is like a room in a large house. At a young age we learn that whenever we enter certain rooms, we are rejected by those from whom we most need acceptance. As a result, we learn simply not to enter those rooms, and by the time we've grown to adulthood we've forgotten they're even there.

It was Carl Jung who first used the word "shadow" to refer to those parts of our personality that we have rejected due to fear, ignorance or shame. His basic premise is simple: "The shadow is the person you would rather not be." He felt that reintegration of these disowned parts of ourselves could have a profoundly positive impact on our emotional and spiritual life. Obviously Jesus felt the same.

We attribute the least acceptable qualities about ourselves to others because we can't face them in ourselves. It isn't always our negative qualities we can't come to terms with, sometimes it's our wonderful qualities. Whether I judge another or engage in hero worship, it's a sure sign I am projecting.

We project onto public figures all the time. Political figures are either lionized or demonized, depending on our point of view. Professional athletes and actors also receive our projections, and are paid handsomely for it. Tiger Woods is a prime example. The public projected its best ideals onto him, but when it became obvious his character wasn't worthy of such adulation, public reaction quickly turned negative.

What happened? Nothing really. He still gets our projections heaped upon him. He got our wonderful parts before; now he gets the ugly parts. It's just the flip side of the same coin. He was never the saint we thought him to be, and he's not the devil incarnate now. He's an imperfect human being, with good parts and bad parts, just like the rest of us. What we think of Tiger Woods says more about us than it does about him. This is the hard truth of projection.

The Tiger Woods saga parallels what happens in our intimate relationships. We fall madly in love, projecting our most beautiful and competent parts onto our partner. All is right with the world. In time however, the polar opposites show up and trouble begins. It's when we project these darker aspects of our nature on our partner that relationships become difficult. It always feels like *they're* the problem, but if we understand the dynamics of projection, we'll know it's time to go inside and learn more about ourselves.

This is an uncomfortable time in a relationship, but also a time of great opportunity. If we take the opportunity to do our inner work, our relationships will blossom. If we don't, we'll keep blaming our partners for things that really have to do with us.

Why Dealing with Our Projections is Difficult

It's hard on our pride. We have to admit that our view of reality might not be quite correct. It's enough of a leap to suggest the labels I attach to people might be wrong, but to suggest that they somehow apply to *me* is a hard pill to swallow.

We have to let go of our judgments. Let's be honest, judging others is fun. One reason we like it so much is that it allows us to feel superior. We come off just a little (or a lot) more moral, hard working, or honest than they are. And that feels good. We all love to be right, and when we judge others we're *always* right—at least in our own eyes.

Our self-image takes a blow when we have to admit we aren't quite the person we thought we were. Most of us aren't afraid to acknowledge our superficial flaws, but owning those we're embarrassed about is something else entirely.

It forces us to deal with our fears. Whenever we think about entering those forgotten rooms, the same childhood fears surface that caused us not to go there in the first place. The rewards are high when we go, but it's still an emotionally difficult place. It's a lot easier to focus on what's wrong with everybody else.

The Benefits of Dealing with Our Projections

It increases self-awareness. This is a benefit in every area of life. When we see ourselves more clearly, we see the world through a less distorted lens. When we are more at peace with ourselves, life flows more smoothly regardless of our circumstances. As we feel more at ease with ourselves, everyone feels more at ease being around us.

Our capacity for intimacy increases. With each room we re-open, more of us is available for life. Our spiritual life improves, as do our marriages and our friendships because there is more of us to give to God, our spouses, and our friends.

It's always a benefit to lose our illusions, even the pleasant ones. A distorted self-image is never a benefit, even when it feels good. It's never comfortable to have our self-image diminished, but it's only our *false* self-image that takes the hit. It's a shock at first, much like jumping into cold water. But once you get used to it, the water's fine.

When we stop blaming others for our discomfort, we take responsibility for our actions and attitudes. Even if we're not proud of them, this is a more powerful platform from which to live our lives. We get more points for being honest with ourselves than we do for perfect behavior. Only our egos tell us otherwise.

It puts us on the positive side of the judgment/compassion scale. We cannot mentally whip someone else without feeling the sting of the lash on some level ourselves. Every judgment of another is essentially a self-judgment—and the same is true of compassion. Many theologians and philosophers would say that finding compassion for ourselves is the main purpose of life. When I can find it for another, I automatically have it for myself.

How Do We Know if We're Projecting?

When the level of our irritation is out of proportion to the "crime," it's a good bet we're projecting. It's not what we see in others that gives us away; it's the charge of our reaction to it. If we just notice, we're probably seeing clearly. If it irritates us, we're probably projecting.

Debbie Ford, author of *The Dark Side of the Light Chasers,* likens it to having electrical outlets on our chest. When we see behavior we cannot face in ourselves, it's like the other person plugs into it. When we realize that we are at least *capable* of the same behavior, it's like covering the socket with a cover plate. We just notice others' behavior. It no longer "plugs us in."

You know you're getting somewhere when you begin to see your irritations as having something to teach you and as an opportunity to find wholeness. You know you're getting nowhere when you continually see them as a nuisance you would just as soon avoid.

Well Worth the Effort

If you're not familiar with the concept of projection, it may take a little time to wrap your head around. Debbie Ford's *The Dark Side of the Light Chasers,* and Byron Katie's *Loving What Is* are both wonderful guides if you wish to begin this process. It takes courage, but nothing will help you understand your partner—and yourself—more.

Once you start working on your projections, seemingly intractable relationship issues begin to melt away. Problems aren't solved as much as they *dissolve,* seemingly on their own. It's a hard truth that those who irritate us are only mirroring a part of ourselves, but when we come to terms with it, it catapults us to another level of life entirely. Our relationships grow immensely because our favorite targets to project upon are those closest to us. In a very real sense, learning to love them is learning to love ourselves.

Forgiveness

It's impossible to be in a successful long-term relationship without forgiveness. When you don't forgive, small things build up over time, and the person you were once so much in love with now seems strangely distant. One day you wake up and realize the magic is gone. Quite often neither partner even knows how it happened. What's worse, neither of you realize that with a little work you can get it back. Love doesn't die—it just gets buried.

The biggest problem with forgiveness is that it's difficult. But why is it so difficult? And does it have to be? As with so many things, maybe we just need to think about it differently.

Forgiveness is closely related to our judgments and projections. Where we are whole, we find it easy to forgive—or more correctly, we don't feel the need to judge in the first place. Projection teaches us that it's only where we are wounded ourselves that we judge others. Unforgiveness is nothing more than a judgment we refuse to let go.

When viewed in this light, it becomes clear why forgiveness is so difficult: we've been going about it wrong. Forgiveness isn't something we do. It's about undoing something (a judgment) we've already done. Forgiveness isn't an action; it's non-action. It isn't something to be accomplished; it's about letting go. If we've found forgiveness difficult, it's because we've been trying to do something that can't be done by trying. Forgiveness is about shifting our mental state, not trying harder. As we learn to let go, forgiveness happens naturally.

A meditation practice can help us forgive because meditation is about learning how to let go. You don't have to bring a specific grievance to mind in order to let it go because meditation is about letting everything go. Our thoughts about the offense and the offender are automatically set aside along with everything else. Meditation also helps us to stay focused on the present moment. If we are fully in the present, we have forgiven by definition because resentment is all about the past.

The principles of imagery also explain why trying to forgive doesn't work. It's never a good idea to bring to mind what you don't want. When you actively try to forgive, the first thing that comes to mind is the offense. This embeds the experience deeper into your psyche; it doesn't get rid of it. It's negative imagery—the old "don't think of an elephant" concept. The intention is good. It's just never works.

At the end of the day, forgiveness is about not putting anyone out of your heart. If you look hard enough for a reason not to, you can usually find one. When you focus on our common humanity, compassion is a lot easier to come by. The more you understand how connected we are, the harder it is to hold a grudge against anyone.

You don't have to chase down every grievance, wrestle it to the ground and beat it into submission with forgiveness. You just have to find a reason to have compassion for your offender. Don't focus on what they did. Just try to find some understanding. What circumstances might have led them to do such a thing? What hardships might they be dealing with? Mentally at least, try walking a mile in their shoes. It will give you a different perspective.

Why We Need to Forgive

The most pragmatic reason to forgive is that **resentment hurts us more than it does them.** The word resent is derived from the Latin prefix, *re-* which means, "again." and *sentire,* which means, "to feel." If the original offense was hurtful, the replays will be too. If the experience was unpleasant the first time, why would we want to feel it again?

Continually replaying an emotionally traumatic experience in our minds, or rehearsing a judgment we hold toward someone, is like a "dog returning to its vomit." It sounds revolting because physiologically it is. With each rehearsal we flood ourselves with the same harmful stress hormones that were originally present. The event is over and done with, but through our mental imagery we keep reliving it. It's been said that refusing to forgive is like us drinking poison and expecting *the other person* to die.

Holding onto resentment **blocks the flow of energy in and around our bodies**. This has mental, emotional, *and* physical consequences. Setting ourselves up as judge, jury, and mental executioner is clearly something we were not designed to do.

The longer we hold a grudge, the more likely we are to seek revenge. Revenge is sweet, but so is breaking into a candy store and eating all the candy. The rush and the sense of power are temporary, and ultimately illusory. A few hours later when we're sitting in our jail cell with a stomachache, we may wonder if it was worth it.

If we don't forgive others, we won't forgive ourselves. Because everyone and everything is interconnected, there is essentially no difference between forgiving them and forgiving ourselves. When we learn to let others off the hook, we automatically let ourselves off too. Thus, forgiveness is one of the greatest self-care tools we have.

Have I Forgiven, or Haven't I?

One thing about forgiveness is certain: just because you *say* you've forgiven, doesn't mean you have. If you find yourself saying, "I'll forgive, but I won't forget," it's doubtful you've forgiven. This statement almost always has an edge to it, and it's the emotional charge that gives us away. As always, it's not what we say that matters, but what we feel.

If you feel the need to make a formal announcement that you've forgiven, then you probably haven't. Forgiveness is a private matter between you and yourself. If you've forgiven in your heart, there's no need to tell anyone about it, least of all the person you've forgiven. Only pride needs to make an announcement. Humility is happy to keep it to itself.

If thoughts about the offense or your offender take up a disproportionate amount of your mental energy, you haven't forgiven. If you find yourself avoiding the person, if you tighten up in their presence, or if you can't look them in the eye, you haven't forgiven.

You can know you have forgiven if you just don't think about it anymore, and if there is no emotional charge when the memory comes to mind. It no longer seems worth it to keep going over the matter. When you have the sense that your mental energies would be better spent elsewhere, you've forgiven—even if you've never uttered the word.

Forgiveness does *not* mean that you allow yourself to be abused or continually taken advantage of. This is not self-care. Take whatever protective steps you need to, then mentally move on. Forgiveness means not reliving hurtful events. It doesn't mean you allow them to continue.

A Gift We Give Ourselves

The table below highlights differences between resentment and forgiveness:

Resentment	Forgiveness
based on judgment	based on grace
ego centered	heart centered
separates us from others	connects us to others
focuses on the past	focuses on the present
results in stuck energy	enhances energy flow
reopens old wounds	heals old wounds
limits our perspective	expands our perspective

The Importance of Healthy Relationships

The preceding comparison makes it clear that forgiveness is something we do for ourselves. It's like periodically changing our oil to get rid of the contaminants we pick up on the road of life. Or taking a shower every morning to wash off yesterday's dirt. The effects of chronic resentment are the same as not changing our oil or not bathing regularly—our vehicles break down, and others don't want to be around us because we smell bad.

Perhaps all that needs to be said on the subject of forgiveness concerns the first thing on the list: Grace is always better than judgment. It feels better, it makes our physiology happier—and it smells better. No matter what the offense, or how hurtful, it's best to let it go.

To Sum Up

All relationships are full of challenges. That's just the way life is. But if you learn how to listen effectively, deal with your projections, and practice forgiveness, your intimate relationships will soar to levels you never dreamed possible. This can have a profoundly positive impact on your health.

Working on these skills will improve any relationship even if it's good already. Each will increase your ability to be fully present with your partner, which is the very definition of intimacy. They will be of benefit even if you are not presently in a romantic relationship. People who listen well, don't blame others for their own issues, and forgive easily are rarely socially isolated.

Regardless of breast cancer, relationship work should be a high priority. It is the best prevention, and if you have cancer already, the best treatment. It is self-care of the highest order. To search out the best in medical care, and give no care to what goes on at home simply doesn't make sense. ॐ

12

Spirit and Your Health

૭

Forgiveness and judgments are traditionally considered spiritual matters. That we find ourselves discussing them as practical ways to enhance our relationships brings us to the subject of how spiritual matters relate to our health.

Eastern medical philosophy considers it self-evident that when we deny our spiritual nature, disease and illness naturally follow, an idea that is outside the Western medical paradigm. Along with the mind-body connection, our spiritual nature is all but denied in the practice of modern medicine.

This strictly material view of the human body has led to some astonishing technological advances, but it has come at a price. In a sense, Western medicine has gained the world but lost its soul. According to Larry Dossey, M.D., a leading advocate of prayer in medicine, "Skirting the spiritual has had a shattering effect on every aspect of contemporary existence."

In his book, *The Art of Compassion,* the Dalai Lama describes two levels of reality. The reality we perceive with our senses and interpret as the real world he calls "conventional reality." "Ultimate reality," on the other hand, is invisible; it is reality we can neither see, hear, touch, taste, nor smell.

Chapter Twelve

Over 90% of people in the United States say they believe in God, but the overwhelming majority of those spend their lives on the plane of conventional reality alone. This reflects a mental separation between the two planes, a condition deeply embedded in the Western psyche. There *is* no separation between the two, of course. The material is simply one aspect of the spiritual. Spirit may be difficult to pin down from a material point of view, but it's no less real than your gallbladder.

In this chapter we will explore the role of prayer in healing, as well as how the spiritual virtues of faith, hope, and love are related to our health. These three form the core of one of the most quoted scriptures in the Christian New Testament:

And now these three remain: faith, hope, love. But the greatest of these is love. (1 Corinthians 13:13 NIV)

Keep in mind that spirituality is not the same as religion. Religion is man's way of organizing spiritual practices. Spirit is what gives religion its life, but the two are not the same. Religious paradigms are some of the most rigid—and the most dangerous. In a sense, religion can be seen as the box we try to fit God into. Spirit can happily exist in a religious box, but by definition cannot be limited to it, which for some reason tends to make people *very* angry.

Religion without Spirit becomes dogma. Spiritual teacher Dan Dierdorff warns that "Once you step in dogma, it's hard to get it off your shoe," which probably tells us all we need to know about the subject. My purpose in this chapter is not to tell you what to believe. Only that what you believe has important implications for your health—and your life.

Prayer

Those who pray regularly don't pay much attention to research studies on prayer. To them such research is like trying to mathematically prove the sun comes up every morning—it's much ado about nothing. People committed to prayer are not impressed with studies showing that prayer works; nor are they discouraged by studies showing otherwise. They just keep on praying.

Still, it can be valuable to know there are studies on prayer, between fifty and seventy-five percent of them showing prayer to have a positive effect.[1,2] We live in an analytical, left-brained society, and it's comforting to know there's proof of what our hearts suspected all along.

Larry Dossey, M.D. catalogs over 130 studies showing the positive effect of prayer in his book, *Healing Words*.[3] Patients being prayed for typically have a shorter duration of illness, leave the hospital sooner, have fewer complications—and occasionally experience the miraculous. There's more scientific evidence that prayer works than there is showing the positive effect of Vitamin C on the common cold.[4]

It seems to matter little who's doing the praying. Studies have been done using energy healers, Christians, Buddhists, and Muslims. Neither does it seem to matter how they pray. Some pray elaborate prayers for healing, others pray a simple, "Thy will be done." Others use no words at all, but simply hold a healing intention in their minds.

There are well-documented health benefits for the pray-er as well as for the one being prayed for. People who attend regular religious services and practice what they believe, including prayer, have lower blood pressure, lower cancer rates, live longer, are less addicted to drugs or alcohol, and cope with chronic disease better.[5]

Chapter Twelve

Clearly, spiritual belief has a healing effect. In fact, a lack of spiritual belief can be as bad for your health as smoking and drinking alcohol.[6] Jim Gordon's quite pragmatic advice on intercessory prayer is, "Go ahead and pray for others; it's good for you. And it just might heal them anyway."

The best proof there is value in prayer may be that we've been doing it in one form or another as long as humankind has existed. If it *never* worked, the practice would have died out long ago. No one keeps up a useless exercise forever.

What is Prayer?

Not surprisingly, something as ethereal as prayer can be difficult to define. Certainly it's broader in scope than the traditional Western view in which we direct our prayers to an old (Caucasian) man in flowing robes sitting on a cloud, who prefers to hear prayers in English. This traditional view of prayer *is* prayer, of course, but it's far from all-inclusive.

Prayer has been defined as opening our hearts and communicating in some way with a power greater than ourselves. When we try to be more concrete than that, we begin leaving things out. The language prayer is spoken in can't possibly matter, and words themselves aren't necessary or mute people could not pray. Most feel that as long as love, compassion, and deep caring are present, there are few other requirements.

It's quite possible that compassion is the only requirement. Whatever words you say without it are unlikely to avail much. And whatever words you add to it may not matter. Compassion itself may *be* the prayer. Like any spiritual practice, prayer has more to do with the intention of the heart than it does anything else.

Of course we know prayer doesn't always work, at least not from our human perspective. If half to three-quarters of studies show a benefit, then one-quarter to half show no benefit at all. Again, to those who pray, this news is like "Dog Bites Man." Those who pray regularly already know sometimes it doesn't work the way they'd like it to. Many people who are prayed for do not recover despite prayers for healing. The fact that we invariably offer up prayers to eradicate illness guarantees that many of them won't be answered. We all have to die of something eventually, no matter how much we pray otherwise.

On a larger scale, a 100% success rate in prayer would certainly wreak global havoc. In the movie *Bruce Almighty*, actor Jim Carrey gets to be God for a week. To save time in answering the vast number of prayers that come in on his computer, Carrey pushes the "yes to all" button. Rioting ensues when millions win the lottery, but win only seventeen dollars each. For reasons we cannot understand, prayer is not a "yes to all" phenomenon.

Praying for someone's healing is much like stepping up to the plate in baseball. As the batter, you're going to miss the ball fairly often. But as long as you keep on swinging, who knows what might happen? You won't hit a home run every time, but if you don't swing the bat you'll *never* hit one.

Prayer Makes Sense

All things considered, it only makes sense to add prayer to whatever else you are doing for your health. It may not work 100% of the time, but neither do surgery and chemotherapy. Herbert Benson considers prayer "as crucial a weapon in our total medical arsenal as antibiotics." After reviewing the research on prayer, Dossey concluded that *not* praying for his patients would be "the equivalent of deliberately withholding a potent drug or surgical procedure."

This is not to advise you to forego medical treatment in lieu of prayer alone. Miraculous healings do occur, but they're rare. This is to say, however, that if you are undergoing conventional medical treatment and not praying in conjunction with it, you may be leaving a lot on the table. Medical treatment is often the method by which prayer is answered. Doing one and not the other is like going out to dig a well, and when someone offers you a shovel, telling them "No thanks, I'll just use my hands."

Despite its documented healing effects, the primary reason to focus on prayer may have nothing to do with our health. That we, in partnership with something greater than ourselves, can pray and effect meaningful change in the world—without ever lifting a finger—says something profound about the human experience. Yes, prayer can improve our condition and occasionally heal us altogether, but to focus on it exclusively as a tool to improve our health is to miss the larger point.

Prayer is a "non-local event," which means it operates outside the space-time continuum. Time and distance do not limit prayer in any way. The prayers your grandparents prayed for you are as much in effect today as they were the day they prayed them. The fact that such a tool is at our disposal whenever we want should give us pause—and hope.

Hope

Hope, which can be defined as a positive expectation of the future, is the baseline necessary for human existence. If you can't see at least the possibility of brighter days ahead, why go on at all? The word "despair" is derived from Latin roots meaning literally, "without hope."

Spirit and Your Health

The Hebrew word for hope is related to the words "cord" and "lifeline." When times are tough, it's hope that allows us to hang on. Hope is the primary antidote to depression, and the ultimate cure for suicide. As long as we have hope, we have a chance. When we lose it, we have no chance at all.

Hope is our ability to see a brighter future. It acts as a counter-balance to our fears, which are negative expectations of the future. Without hope, our fears would soon overwhelm us. Hope might also be called optimism or positivity. Optimism and pessimism are simply two different ways of looking at life. Martin Seligman, author of *Learned Optimism*, calls them our "explanatory style," which he defines as the manner in which we explain to ourselves why events happen.[7]

We already know everyone does not perceive the same event in the same way. The difference, therefore, is in the perceiver, not that which is perceived. Whether the glass is half empty or half full is a matter of how we look at it, not of how much water there is. And by and large, how we look at it is learned.

Contrary to popular belief, there is no optimism gene. Which means if we're pessimists, we don't have to stay that way. Seligman titled his book *Learned Optimism* precisely because optimism is a skill that can be acquired with practice. Acquiring it is more important than we might think. Whether we are optimistic or pessimistic affects our health almost as clearly as do physical factors, as evidenced by the following facts:[8]

- Optimists have half the rate of infections as pessimists
- Optimists visit the doctor half as much as pessimists
- Optimists have better health habits than pessimists
- Optimists have stronger immune systems
- Optimists tend to live longer

Chapter Twelve

Breast cancer patients who have an optimistic explanatory style survive longer than women who describe themselves as feeling helpless and resigned to a negative outcome.[9,10,11] The Irish proverb would seem to be true: Hope is the physician of every misery.

The relatively new science of Psychoneuroimmunology (PNI) shows quite clearly that our mental and emotional state directly affects our immune system. In a landmark study on the subject, a group of rats were exposed to electric shocks from which they could not escape.[12] Nothing they did mattered; the electric shocks came anyway.

As the rats learned they were helpless, they grew visibly listless and their immune systems began to fail. They grew more tumors and experienced more infections. In other words, *their immune systems mirrored their external behavior.* They died much sooner than the rats exposed to electric shocks they could take some action to avoid.

The parallels between this study and the modern medical breast cancer paradigm are unmistakable. Pinning breast cancer "causation" on genetics alone takes away any hope you might have of doing something to avoid it. Taking away this hope causes women to be passive in terms of prevention. But the passivity isn't warranted by the facts, and may itself be harmful.

It should be clear by now that you are not hopeless (powerless) in the face of breast cancer. We've discussed much you can do to decrease your risk, and there's more to come. If you allow yourself to be influenced by current medical thinking, however, you aren't likely to do any of it, since you'll have no reason to believe it will matter.

Hope doesn't guarantee a positive outcome, but it does guarantee the possibility of one, which is all anyone can ask. Hope knows your choices are important. It's a splash of water in the face to wake us up from the culture-induced illusion that nothing we do matters. *Everything* we do matters. Believing it may matter most of all.

Faith

Now faith is being sure of what we hope for, and certain of what we do not see. (Hebrews 11:1 NIV)

Prior to becoming president, Barak Obama wrote a book titled *The Audacity of Hope* in which he defines hope as a dogged optimism about the future. Hope, like everything else, is a spectrum ranging from a type of wishful thinking, to a more confident optimism about the future.

As the above scripture verse indicates, when hope becomes so dogged it seems real, we call it faith. Faith is so sure of what we hope for it seems like reality now. Faith is the next step on the ladder. Faith is built on hope. It contains hope. You can't have faith without hope. But faith is greater than hope. It's hope that's gone to the gym and worked out.

Faith is the word we use to describe our relationship to the invisible realm. Our level of faith tells us whether our main focus is based in material reality or in ultimate reality. Are we stuck on the surface of life, reacting to what we see with our physical eyes, or can we "see" something deeper?

In our culture, when we speak about faith, it is generally understood to be spiritual faith, or faith in God. But faith is not limited to spiritual issues. We can have faith in anything. We can have faith in ourselves, faith in our country, faith in our job, or faith in our friends. When we worry, we are showing faith in our fears. Technically speaking, when someone says they have faith, the question must be asked, "Faith in what?"

Chapter Twelve

Faith is part of the human design, and each of us is endowed with a measure of it. Faith contains enormous power. It's just a matter of how we choose to invest that power. Investing our faith wisely means having more faith in our hopes than we do our fears.

Another word for faith is belief. Quite simply, our world is defined by what we believe. The voice of Hope and the voice of Fear speak to us, mostly through the images in our minds. In any given situation, we will always "hear" both voices. Which we choose to believe will determine what we experience.

It's a replay of our discussion on stress. It seems like some events affect us adversely while others have a more positive effect. But in truth, it's what we *believe* about those events that determines how they affect us. It seems we have more power than we give ourselves credit for.

The Placebo Effect

The power of our belief to heal lies hidden right before our eyes, masquerading as the placebo effect. As most are aware, a placebo is a sugar pill (or the equivalent), given to a patient who is told they are receiving the real medicine. As it happens, many who get the sugar pill get better, even though the pill clearly has no therapeutic effect. Often they show the same improvement as those who took the real medicine

The word placebo is a Latin word meaning "I will please." It is related to our word "placate." It has a negative connotation in medical circles, implying a sense of fakery. In medical thought, the placebo is equivalent to something false. "Sure, the patients get better, but it isn't real. It's all in their head."

True, it is in their head, but it isn't *only* in their head. The physical improvements patients get from the placebo effect are indistinguishable from those achieved by the actual drug. The astonishing fact is, for *any* disease state, and for *any* treatment, roughly 35 percent of patients show improvement due the placebo effect alone.[13] Sometimes the percentage is higher.

Placebo surgery has even been shown to be effective. A 2003 study at Baylor University showed that patients who underwent arthroscopic knee surgery had no better results than those who simply went to the operating room, and under general anesthesia, had small surgical incisions in their knee similar to those of the actual surgery.[14] The patients receiving the placebo surgery fared no worse and no better than patients who received the real treatment.

The deeper implications of the placebo effect are staggering. If it isn't the pill or the surgery that makes patients better, what is it? The inescapable conclusion is that the patients get better because they *believe* they will get better. There is no external cause for the patients' improvement. Rather, the placebo effect is an outward manifestation of an internal cause—namely the patients' belief. Placebo tells us that, at least in part, faith in the therapy *is* the therapy.

Understood correctly, the placebo effect is a gateway to our deeper selves. It touches on the interplay between our reliance on an infinite God to heal us, and our responsibility to use the innate power that same infinite God gave us to heal ourselves.

At the present time the placebo effect is strictly used in pharmaceutical research. In order to prove the efficacy of a new drug, it must be shown to have a therapeutic effect over and above the placebo effect. If it does, it is deemed effective. If it doesn't, it's back to the drawing board. From the medical perspective placebo is no more than a nuisance, adding time and expense to the testing of new pharmaceuticals.

Placebo is a doorway to a new realm of healing possibilities, but we can't expect a pharmaceutical-based medical system to recognize its value any time soon. Seen clearly, placebo would be self-defeating to that system. In a self-care paradigm, however, taking advantage of the placebo effect is a no-brainer. It is a reality we can't wake up to soon enough.

According to Elizabeth Kuby, author of *Faith and the Placebo Effect*, herself a breast cancer survivor who was healed without conventional medical therapy:

> The medicine of the future will concentrate on triggering placebo effects. Encouraging patients to have faith in their ability to cure themselves will produce more cures than are dreamed of in our present medical philosophy. Doctors will be doctors of the spirit. "What about science?" you ask. This *is* science. It's the science that science has not yet caught up with.[15]

But before that happens, we'll probably have to change the name. The associations between placebo and trickery are too strong. I like the term "Inner Physician" because that's exactly what the placebo effect demonstrates. Our Inner Physician, when fully unleashed, is capable of the miraculous.

The only problem we have with the process is that it takes place beneath our conscious, reasoning mind. As long as our intellect is king we seriously handicap our Inner Physician. For most, the conscious mind must be fooled in order to unlock the placebo effect. But with increasing awareness and a little practice, this needn't always be the case.

The Nocebo Effect

Unfortunately, the power of our belief works not only in the positive, but also in the negative. In other words, our negative expectations can be as harmful as our positive expectations are healing. The negative aspect of the equation has been called the nocebo effect. Nocebo comes from the Latin word meaning "I shall harm." It is placebo's evil twin.

If placebo is an opportunity missed, nocebo is a danger unrecognized. Some of the greatest harm we do as physicians is unwittingly setting up patients for negative outcomes by quoting survival statistics without explaining how they were derived and the uncertainties that surround them.

Patients told they have six months to live will often do exactly that. In *The Biology of Belief,* Bruce Lipton relates the case of a man with esophageal carcinoma given six months to live, who died exactly six months later even though his tumor was far too small to have killed him.[16] At autopsy, no cause of death was found.

It's hard for those steeped in the medical perspective to believe nocebo can have such a deadly effect, but it clearly can. It is a well-known phenomenon that some people die when bitten by non-poisonous snakes they believed to be poisonous. Being "frightened to death" is not just an old saying.

Unfortunately for us, our negative expectations don't know the difference between a snake and a poor prognosis. Just like our positive beliefs, they seek out what they're "aimed" at. And if they are aimed at a poor outcome, the effect will be harmful—sometimes to the extreme.

The nocebo effect is one of the hidden dangers in the modern explosion of genetic testing and breast cancer risk assessment. When considering any high-risk statistic that has been applied to you, it is extremely important to keep nocebo in mind. Because it lies outside the medical paradigm, it's unlikely your doctor will be thinking about it when he or she talks to you. But for your own good, you *have* to think about it. A label of "high risk" or "poor prognosis" is a potentially deadly seed planted into your subconscious.

Nocebo is subtle, powerful, and occasionally fatal. And it

doesn't always kill quickly—it can kill slowly over time. There is an old Russian proverb that describes this truth: "The mind is capable of holding a conversation with the body that ends in death."

How might nocebo affect you? No one knows. It's likely that some will be affected more strongly than others, but it is impossible to know what that means for you. The only thing you can do is to be aware of it, and work to keep your fears and negative expectations from getting the better of you. Keep your expectations positive. It's the best protection.

Placebo and nocebo are opposite sides of the same coin. In a sense, they both tell us the same thing—our faith is powerful. Powerful enough to heal us, and powerful enough to harm us. So invest your belief wisely, in areas that benefit you, not in areas that act to your detriment. If you are at high risk for developing breast cancer, believe more in what you can do to lower your risk than you do in the risk itself. If you're a survivor or are currently struggling with the disease, believe more in your health than you do your disease. It will make a difference. It could make all the difference.

Love

Most would find it intuitively obvious that "love is the greatest of these." Hope, faith, and love are sequential steps on the ladder of life. Hope keeps us in the game; faith is how we play; love is how we win. Faith and hope are powerful, but love is much, much more. But what *is* love? The word is so misused in modern culture it can be hard to know.

If I love my wife, but I also love ice cream and watching football, what does that say about love? And how is it supposed to make my wife feel? She might legitimately want to know where she falls on the list. Is it first on anniversaries and birthdays, but somewhere else when it's Sunday afternoon or time for dessert?

When it comes to defining love, perhaps more than with any other spiritual virtue, the words get in the way. The New Testament gets at it better by using different words for love (at least in the original Greek) and by not using the term love to refer to our attachment to material objects. In the Greek there is a clear distinction between *phileo*, which refers to fondness, and *agape*, which is the unconditional love Jesus spoke about.

Unconditional love can be thought of as love without an object. It's something that resides within us and radiates outward, not something we bestow on a favored few. It's a state of being, not a commodity. If I love someone because of "this," and hate someone else because of "that," it is certain my feelings are due to my own projections. If I need a reason to love someone—it isn't love.

Russell Targ, author of *Limitless Mind*, puts it this way: "It may be hard to imagine, but the significant love available to us transcends girlfriends, boyfriends, romance, or sex. The love I'm talking about exists at our core. If you are vigilant, no one can ever separate you from that love."

This is the type of love that transcends circumstances and is unconcerned with character flaws. It is the divinity within each of us. It isn't something we need to search for. At the deepest level, it is who we are. It can never be found "out there," because it's already "in here." Thus, we can only uncover it by going within.

There is a clear interplay between meditation and love. The mind, when it is quiet and open, has the opportunity to be overwhelmed by love. Buddhists call this "undifferentiated awareness." This is the deep awareness that there are no real boundaries between any of us. This naturally leads to our undeniable relationship to the Infinite.

Chapter Twelve

Love and the Heart

For thousands of years nearly every culture on earth has considered the heart as the seat of our emotions and the place love originates. Modern science shows that this is not just metaphorical. The anatomy and physiology of the heart is far more complex than we previously suspected. There's a reason love and other strong emotions are perceived in the center of the chest, and it's solidly grounded in the structure and function of the heart.

The research done in this area by the Institute of HeartMath is nothing short of remarkable.[17] It brings together modern science and ancient philosophy, making scientific sense of what once could only be found in spiritual texts.

Conventional medicine views the heart as a simple pump that functions under the direction of the brain. It does, of course, but like everything else, it works both ways. Communication between the heart and the brain is a dynamic, two-way dialogue in which one organ continually influences the other.

The heart communicates with the brain not only by means of neurological pathways, but also by the interaction of electromagnetic fields. The latter, called cardio-electromagnetic communication, has been shown to affect the brain's electrical activity and performance.

Each organ in the body generates its own electromagnetic field, the body's overall field being a summation of them all. The heart is the most powerful generator of electromagnetic energy in the body, producing the largest magnetic field of any organ including the brain.

The heart's electrical field is 60 times greater in amplitude that the brain's, and its magnetic field is 5,000 times greater in strength. The heart field can be detected several feet away from the body in all directions. (Fig. 1) It is important to note that the brain's electromagnetic field functions *within* the cardiac field.

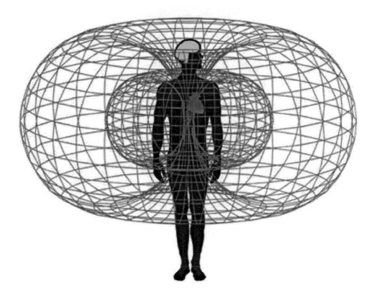

The Heart's Magnetic Field
(fig. 1)
[with permission. Institute of HeartMath]

The cardiac field is constantly changing, and is affected by our emotional states. Positive emotional states such as love and appreciation strengthen the cardiac field, while negative emotions such as anger and rage diminish it. A spectral analysis of an electrocardiogram (ECG) shows that the electrical activity of the heart is more coherent when we feel appreciation than when we are frustrated, coherence being defined as electrical activity working in greater harmony. (Fig. 2)

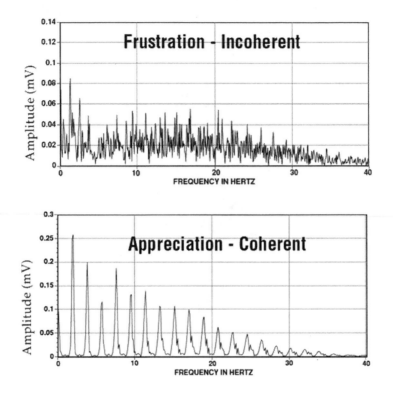

Spectral analysis of an electrocardiogram
(ECG) during appreciation and frustration.

(fig. 2)

[with permission. Institute of HeartMath]

When the cardiac field is strong, what is referred to as an "open heart," mental functioning is optimal. We have greater clarity, awareness, *and* increased cognitive function. Not only does the brain function better, the entire body does. When our hearts are filled with compassion, every organ in our body functions at a higher level. Some say the purpose of negative emotions is simply to alert us that our cardiac field is weakening.

Understanding the power of living from the heart can literally change the way we think about life. The HeartMath research makes it clear that being in a positive emotional state is in our own best interest. It is the most effective—and the healthiest—way to go through life. Compassion, as it turns out, makes good physiologic sense.

Love positively affects our relationships, goes hand in hand with an optimistic outlook, and indicates a healthy processing of emotions—all of which are associated with increased survival in cancer patients. But we're beyond the question of cancer here. We're into the realm of how we as humans were designed to function optimally. Novelist Henry Miller says, "The goal of life is not to possess power, but to radiate it." This can only be done with an open heart.

Love is the fabric of the universe. It is the power underlying everything. Our judgments and projections separate us from it. Only unbridled compassion opens our hearts, allowing us to tap into it. What is unbridled compassion? It is compassion that excludes no one—not even ourselves.

Whether you call it unconditional love, undifferentiated awareness, or an open heart doesn't matter. What matters is that you access it and live from it. Love is a discipline, a practice, and a way of life. It is a commitment we make to live a certain way—no matter what. It's not easy to do, but the rewards for trying are high. Love is the fuel for everything good in our lives. It pays to keep our tank as full as we possibly can.

Love ties everything together—and simplifies it. Despite all their disagreements, every religion in the world agrees on this: God *is* Love. One could make the argument that when it gets more complicated than that things start to break down.

Chapter Twelve

Pierre Teilhard de Chardin, an early 20th century French philosopher, had this to say about love: "Someday, after he has tamed the wind and the waves and gravity, man will harness for God the power of love, and then, for the second time in the history of the world, he will have discovered fire."

All you need to know about what love is, what it asks of us, and the powerful effect it has on others, is contained in the following piece written by Dr. Richard Selzer, describing an experience he had with a patient and her husband.[18]

I stand by the bed where a young woman lies, her face postoperative, her mouth twisted in palsy, clownish. A tiny twig of the facial nerve, the one to the muscles of her mouth, has been severed. She will be thus from now on. As surgeon, I had followed with religious fervor the curve of her flesh, I promise you that. Nevertheless, to remove the tumor in her cheek, I had to cut the little nerve.

Her young husband is in the room. He stands on the opposite side of the bed, and together they seem to dwell in the evening lamplight, isolated from me, private. "Who are they," I ask myself, "he and this wry mouth who gaze and touch each other so generously?"

"Will my mouth always be like this?" she asks. "Yes," I say. "It is because the nerve was cut." She nods, is silent. But the young man smiles. "I like it," he says. "It's kind of cute."

All at once I know who he is. I understand, and I lower my gaze. One is not bold in an encounter with a god. Unmindful of my presence, he bends to kiss her crooked mouth, and I'm so close I can see how he twists his own lips to accommodate hers, to show her that their kiss still works.

I remember that the gods appeared in ancient Greece as mortals, and I hold my breath and let the wonder in. &

13

Risk Revisited

❦

Now that we've explored the concept of self-care—mind, body, and spirit—it's time to take another look at breast cancer risk and survival statistics. Considering all we have learned up to now, it's time to reassess.

To be brief and to the point, nobody knows what the breast cancer risk is for someone who undergoes a comprehensive program of self-care as outlined in this book.

Those who undertake a multi-pronged approach aimed at improving the nutritional, emotional, physical, mental, relational, and spiritual aspects of their health are simply off the charts. No research study exists that has ever asked the question.

The same is true for survival statistics. The women in Dr. Spiegel's study doubled their expected survival time simply by being in a group, with no change in medical therapy. No one's ever studied what would happen to women who participated in a similar group and improved their eating habits, or had people pray for them, or started exercising and lost weight. More to the point, what would happen to survival time in women who did *all* of these?

If you're currently struggling with breast cancer, no matter how advanced, no one knows what's going to happen to you. Don't let anyone make you think your future is certain, because it isn't. If you are actively engaged in your own self-care, you too are in uncharted territory. There are no statistics that apply to you.

Don't ignore risk and survival statistics entirely. They can give you an idea of how high the stakes are for you, and what your margin for error is in undertaking a program of self-care. Just remember that they're ballpark estimates. Once you get the estimate, don't forget how big the ballpark is.

Take these numbers as a general guideline for the average person. Then determine not to be average. They are accurate for large groups of women. They may not be accurate for you. Let the numbers spur you on to a higher degree of self-care. Make them work for you. Don't be a slave to them. Even if you are BRCA positive, your risk can be modified.[1]

For high-risk women and survivors, the uncertainty over risk and survival statistics is good news. It means you aren't stuck in the grim box that well-meaning doctors or sterile statistics may have put you. The first and biggest step in climbing out is to believe that you can. And the most dangerous thing you can do is believe you can't.

A Word about Research

Climbing out of the box begins with seeing through the air of infallibility the culture projects onto medical research. Western medicine prides itself on being evidence-based, meaning that standard practices are based on research. But if research studies are the gold standard, why do they contradict each other so often, and why do the experts argue over them so much? Research is a powerful tool, but it has its shortcomings. Things are rarely as cut and dried as they seem.

Risk Revisited

From the holistic perspective, it's obvious why research studies conflict. Emotional, spiritual, and nutritional factors are rarely taken into account. These factors are so varied and so complex, randomized controlled trials can't get an accurate picture. Some of the most important factors aren't even in the worldview of the researcher. A look at some examples should help clear up why things are so unclear:

The Nurses' Health Study, conducted by researchers at the Harvard School of Public Health, is widely known as the longest running, premier study on women's health.[2] The study began in 1976 and involved over 120,000 nurses across the country. In 1980, a dietary questionnaire was added to the study and the data collected over several decades.

One conclusion of the study was that fruit and vegetable intake made no difference in breast cancer incidence. Those with the highest intake of fruits and vegetables got breast cancer just as often as those with the lowest intake. But as Colin Campbell points out in his critique of the study, the nurses' diets were not controlled for animal protein intake.[3]

As a group, the amount of meat consumed by the nurses in this study was well above the general U.S. population, which is already high by world standards. The amount of meat they ate on a daily basis would "practically qualify them as carnivores." They consumed very low amounts of whole, plant-based foods.

What the study showed, according to Campbell, was that in a large group of women with a high animal protein intake, eating small amounts of fruits and vegetables had no impact on breast cancer incidence. That's a far cry from "fruit and vegetable intake has no effect on breast cancer risk." In Campbell's opinion, the Nurses' Health Study, revered by many, "is the premier example of how reductionism in science can create massive amounts of confusion."

Chapter Thirteen

Another nutritional study published in the Journal of the American Medical Association (JAMA) in 2005 also showed that fruit and vegetable intake had no impact on breast cancer risk.[4] The study compared two groups, one getting 114 grams or less of fruits per day, and another group eating 367 grams or more of fruits a day. The numbers were similar for the vegetable group (<109 grams vs. >309 grams). The study was designed to show whether there was any difference in breast cancer risk between the two groups, which there wasn't. The problem is, this level of daily fruit and vegetable intake is far below recommended guidelines.

A medium apple is approximately 250 grams, meaning that this study compared women eating half a medium apple a day to women eating about one and a half medium apples a day, and a group eating approximately one bell pepper a day with a group eating a bell pepper and two small tomatoes.[5]

In this study, the women who consumed the most fruits and vegetables didn't come close to the recommended 5 to 13 servings of fruits and vegetables a day. This would be akin to studying water consumption in rats by giving a group of rats one drop of water a day, a control group three drops a day, and after observing that all the rats died within a few days, concluding that "Tripling daily water intake in rats has no impact on survival."

Such a study could be described in exactly the same way as the JAMA study: well-executed, statistical results properly calculated, but misleading conclusion due to the design of the study. A more accurate conclusion of the JAMA study might have been: "There is no difference in breast cancer risk between women who eat hardly any fruits and vegetables at all, and women whose fruit and vegetable consumption is slightly higher, but still inadequate."

Wading Through Controversy

These controversies rage back and forth in the medical research world. And it isn't only about eating more fruits and vegetables. Controversy and contradictions can be found everywhere. It makes decision-making complicated and stressful for the average person. Here are a few helpful hints on how to make some sense of it all:

When considering research studies, think risk-benefit ratio rather than hard science. Scientists are constrained by the scientific method. They're looking for factual, reproducible, physical evidence. Researchers must follow rigorous guidelines, both in the design and interpretation of their studies. If they don't, no one will publish their work. But you, as a normal human being, are just trying to make a reasonable decision. You are not, and should not, be constrained by the same things as a research scientist. You're not trying to publish a scientific study, after all. You're just trying to live your life.

Can eating more fruits and vegetables prevent cancer? The overwhelming majority of studies suggest the answer is yes, while others say it won't make any difference. But how risky is eating more fruits and vegetables? Most would find the health benefits of doing so intuitively obvious.

If it might prevent cancer, it isn't going to hurt you, and it's good for you anyway, the most reasonable thing to do is eat more of them. Besides, Mom always told me I should eat more fruits and vegetables, and her advice was free. This is what I call the Mom test: **if the risk is low, the studies disagree, and Mom comes down on one side or the other, always go with what Mom says.**

When you're investigating the research, it's also a good idea to pay attention to how you feel. If you begin to feel helpless, hopeless, or just plain "yuck" as you're reading an article, put it down and don't go back to it, no matter what it says. **If the risk is low, and the**

studies disagree, always go with the one that gives you hope.

If you're at high risk for breast cancer, for instance, and focus on the studies showing that lowering your stress level decreases your risk, you will be encouraged to lower your stress level. But if you focus on those studies showing no effect, it's easier to have the attitude of "why bother?" Hopelessness will kill your energy, your vitality, and maybe even you.

All of the self-care techniques in this book fall into the low-risk category. None of them will hurt you. At worst, you'll be healthier, happier, and more energetic; at best, they may save your life. It's hard to argue with that.

Don't underestimate the power of the paradigm effect. It can skew the (perceived) outcome of research studies more than you think. A prime example is a study of breast cancer risk in identical twins published in 2002.[6] The study showed that if one twin was diagnosed with breast cancer, the lifetime risk in the other twin was 1 in 3. This is triple the risk in the average population.

Accordingly, the initial news release in the U.K. in May, 2002 was titled, "Triple Risk for Breast Cancer Twins." The study was touted as "increasing scientific understanding about the genetics of breast cancer," as well as adding "to a growing number of studies on breast cancer genetics, which are important for increasing knowledge of the disease and tailoring treatments."[7]

Things look differently, however, from another point of view. Three times the risk of the general population is significant, but hardly surprising considering the genetic similarity of twins. One could rightly make the comment, "Tell us something we don't already know." The study was authored, interpreted, and presented to the public through the lens of genetic determinism.

The study is a prime example of the paradigm effect because the same findings can point to *exactly the opposite conclusion* that the author came to. Yes, a 1 in 3 lifetime risk is high. But if 1 out of 3 will go on to develop breast cancer, it means that 2 out of 3 won't—even with identical genes.

To those not steeped in genetic determinism this seems obvious. Why don't the other two-thirds get it? What answer could there possibly be besides environmental and lifestyle factors? The same study, interpreted and publicized differently, could be a clarion call for cancer prevention. "Breast Cancer Not Just a Genetic Disease," would have been just as valid a headline.

The final word on research studies? Let the buyer beware. Don't accept any of them out of hand, even what I present here. Check them out. Shop around. Make sure to look at studies written from different points of view. This is *especially* true on the internet. If the findings conflict, apply all the tests we've just discussed. Trust your own common sense, intuition, and decision-making ability more than you do the experts' opinions. Even if the experts all agree, it doesn't make them right. The world did turn out to be round, after all.

On the Lighter Side

Wading through the research can be like finding your way in a maze. It's hard work, and often confusing. But it can be fun too. Occasionally you run across some pretty amusing things. Like a study showing that women who drink beer have a higher bone density than those who don't.[8] The study noted that both beer drinking and bone density decrease with age.

This seems like a valid observation, but what are we supposed to do with that information, put beer on tap in all the nursing homes? Maybe the two facts aren't even related. Maybe osteoporotic ninety-year-olds just have a harder time getting down to the tavern than they used to.

Then there's the brain mapping study where one of the partici-pants placed their head in a PET scanner while having sex with their partner.[9] The purpose of the study was to see which areas of the brain are active during sexual arousal and orgasm. While this is a perfectly logical way to get such information, I find it difficult to concentrate on the findings.

I keep having visions of hoards of local college students over-powering hospital security and storming the Radiology department to be included in the study. Or imagining the technologist giving the participant pre-scan directions: "Go ahead and have an orgasm when you're ready—but *don't move!*"

Such a study is proof positive that researchers look at things differently than the general population. I'm sure the information on orgasm and brain function is useful on some level, but what most of us want to know is—how *did* they manage that?

Laughter is Good Medicine

We must have been designed to laugh, or it wouldn't be so good for us. Laughter is a natural medicine. Research studies have shown that laughter boosts the immune system, stimulates the heart and lungs, relieves pain, balances blood pressure, and enhances mental function.[10] Laughter is also a great way of moving stuck emotional energy.

Laughter enhances quality of life, improves attitude, and leads to an overall sense of well-being. It can serve as a distraction, offering a brief respite from the more pressing concerns of life. It can be viewed as a mental vacation, because when we're laughing, no other thought can enter our mind. In this sense, laughter is a meditation.

Interest in laughter as therapy began with Norman Cousins'

classic book, *Anatomy of an Illness,* in which he chronicled his healing from a mysterious and painful chronic disease by self-administered intravenous Vitamin C and laughter therapy. "Laughing yourself well" isn't common, but maybe that's because so few have tried it. Cousins clearly proved it's possible.

Laughter may seem incongruous in a book about cancer, but the more serious the issue, sometimes the greater the need for it. Ingrid Betancourt, a former presidential candidate in Columbia, was abducted and held captive for six years in the Columbian jungle. She had this to say about laughter in her book, *Even Silence Has an End:* "I felt intuitively that laughter was the beginning of wisdom, as it was indispensable to survival."

No matter what difficulty you are facing, it's important to keep a place in your heart for laughter. It can make the good days great, and the dark days survivable. No matter what else you lose, never lose your sense of humor. Cry when you need to, but otherwise laugh as much as you can. ❧

14
Understanding Mammography

❧

The controversy surrounding breast cancer doesn't end with risk and prevention issues. It only begins there. Mammography, the most common way for breast cancer to be diagnosed, has its own unique set of controversial issues. Because most women will have a mammogram at some time in their lives, it will be helpful to take a detailed look at the process. The more you know about it, the better. We'll begin by taking a closer look at the controversy over screening mammography guidelines.

The Screening Mammography Controversy

In recent years there has been broad agreement on recommendations for screening mammography: Get a screening mammogram once a year beginning at age 40 for as long as you are reasonably healthy.

In November, 2009, the US Preventive Services Task Force (USPSTF) announced new guidelines recommending *against* women between 40 and 49 getting routine screening mammograms. Women between 50 and 75 should get a mammogram every other year according to the new guidelines, and there was no recommendation either way for women over 75.[1] The guidelines were announced without warning, among much fanfare and media coverage.

Nothing seemed unusual at first. New information comes out all the time and most assumed the new guidelines simply reflected the latest developments in the field. But problems began immediately when it became clear there *was* no new information, and that few agreed with the new recommendations.

Later the same day the American College of Radiology (ACR), and the Society of Breast Imaging (SBI), the professional societies directly involved in screening mammography, came out with statements strongly opposing the new guidelines. The American Cancer Society (ACS), an independent organization, also disagreed. The new guidelines were called "unscientific" and seemed to reflect a "conscious decision to ration care" in the opinion of some breast imaging experts.[2] Shockingly, none of these experts had even been consulted by the USPSTF prior to the announcement.

As it turns out, the USPSTF, a government agency few had heard of until this point, had based its new guidelines on computer models of previous research studies. Most had assumed their findings were based on new information, but there was none. The new guidelines reversed the Task Force's previous recommendation in 2002, which recommended yearly screening mammography beginning at age 40. Many suspected this wasn't about who should get a mammogram, but who was going to pay for it.

In early December, Dr. Ned Calonge, Chairman of the USPSTF's medical arm, was called before Congress to testify because of the uproar caused by the new recommendations. Under scrutiny, Dr. Calonge said the guidelines were "poorly worded" and "didn't say what they (the Task Force) meant them to say."[3] A few days later, the guidelines were revised to state that women between the ages of 40 and 49 should discuss the issue with their doctor and make an individual decision about screening mammography. The recommendation for a mammogram every other year after age 50 was left intact.

In the following months, criticism continued to mount over the controversial new guidelines. In February, 2010, a review of the USPSTF's report methodology was published which found that the report did not meet established standards for systematic reviews.[4]

In April, 2010, Daniel Kopans, M.D., Head of the Breast Imaging Division at the Mass General Hospital, and faculty at Harvard Medical School, denounced the USPSTF guidelines, saying they would "set women's health back more than 20 years and should be rescinded."[5]

The mounting opposition, both in the scientific community and in Congress, had an effect. In July, 2010, new government regulations were announced requiring insurance plans to cover screening mammography according to the Task Force's *2002* guidelines which recommended yearly screening mammography beginning at age 40. The more recent 2009 guidelines were considered "not current."[6]

In October, 2010, President Obama kicked off breast cancer awareness month with a speech in which he recommended women begin screening at age 40 and pledged that yearly mammograms would be covered by insurance plans starting at this age.[7] In an ironic twist, this chapter of the screening mammogram controversy came to an end by the U.S. government repudiating its own guidelines. The media blitz at the beginning, however, was not duplicated at the end. Many women are still confused.

Following the Clues

It can be difficult for a non-medical person to make heads or tails out of such a controversy. When the experts disagree it's very disconcerting for the general public. It's hard to know what you should do, but there are always clues if you look closely.

It was suspicious that the new guidelines came from a government agency in the middle of a health care debate about cutting costs. The initial media blitz touting the new guidelines without any opposing viewpoint was also suspect. And it's unheard of that a professional society has its guidelines changed by an outside agency without even being consulted.

At the time of their decision, no one on the board of USPSTF was actively working in the field of breast cancer diagnosis or treatment. There was no radiologist, no breast surgeon, and no oncologist. The board was mostly made up of family physicians that do not have a clinical practice. A pediatrician and a psychiatric nurse practitioner were also members of the board. No one questions their public health credentials—only their ability to make a balanced decision without input from experts working in the field.

The fact that the new guidelines were based on the Task Force's own computer models using only data they themselves chose to consider is a giant red flag. Well-respected studies from Sweden and the Netherlands, both showing over a forty percent decrease in breast cancer deaths in the screening groups, were not included for consideration, while several questionable studies were included.[8]

The "Age" trial was considered by the Task Force, even though only single view mammography (known to miss 25% of cancers) was employed.[9] A Canadian study was also considered even though women with palpable masses, some of which turned out to be advanced cancers, were included in the screening group.[10,11] Screening mammography, by definition, is for women with no symptoms.

From the outside looking in, it seems that the Task Force's

computer models came up with exactly the answer they expected. One could almost have predicted the outcome without even bothering to run the models. Perhaps the kindest thing that can be said of their findings is that they do not represent a balanced view.

Nor were all of their findings highly publicized. An editorial accompanying the USPSTF guidelines stated that screening mammography every other year between the ages of 50 and 69 would avert 70 to 90 percent of the breast cancer deaths that are averted now with yearly screening. This means that the Task Force was knowingly willing to accept a 10 to 30 percent increase in breast cancer deaths in this age group.

It makes even less sense to deny screening altogether to women under 50. In a country where the breast cancer rate has nearly tripled since World War II, and where cancers are being found at an increasingly younger age, why would we leave this group of women out in the cold?

It's true that cancers are less common in women under 50 than they are in older women, but they're still relatively common. And the cancers in this age group tend to be more aggressive, making the diagnosis of an early cancer that much more valuable.[12] Since widespread screening was introduced in the U.S. in 1990, there has been a 30 percent decrease in breast cancer mortality, *including* the 40-49 age group.[13]

Not offering any early detection to women in this age range doesn't even make financial sense. True, the insurance industry would save a lot of money on mammograms and biopsies, but end-stage cancer treatment is extremely expensive, and the increase in these treatments that would surely follow would easily swallow up the savings.[14,15,16]

Screening mammography is like buying an insurance policy or wearing a seatbelt. You do it not because it's likely that you're house will burn down, or you will be seriously injured in a car accident. You do it because the relative cost of the protection is low and the consequences of the event are potentially devastating.

Statistically, the most likely scenario is that you will have your yearly screening mammograms, perhaps be called back for extra views once or twice in your life, and maybe have to undergo a biopsy, which will most likely be benign. The cost of the mammograms and possible biopsies (all covered by health insurance), along with the emotional distress that can accompany them, will be the price you pay for this insurance.

All insurance works the same way: people are willing to pay the premium if it isn't prohibitive, knowing they'll be covered if the unthinkable happens. What they get most from the insurance is peace of mind, since the unthinkable is an uncommon event. In terms of breast cancer, this means you may have your yearly mammograms, perhaps endure some emotional distress along the way due to a benign biopsy, and the life that is saved may be your sister's, or your neighbor's, or someone you don't even know. It probably *won't* be you, But it could be.

Realizing that mammography is imperfect, and realizing that it comes with the possible cost of a few false alarms, the most telling statistic is this: *The majority of women who die of breast cancer are those who did not have routine yearly mammographic screening.* Seventy-five percent of the deaths occurred in women in this category in a recent analysis of breast cancer deaths in Massachusetts.[17]

Mammography doesn't prevent breast cancer, but it may prevent your *dying* of breast cancer. The thirty percent reduction in breast cancer mortality since 1990 is virtually all due to mammography's ability to diagnose breast cancers as small as a few millimeters, while they're still easily treatable.[18] With few exceptions, small cancers don't kill you—larger ones do.

At the end of the day, screening mammography is a personal choice. Take a look at it from all sides of the issue. Consider the risks, the cost, and the potential benefits, and decide whether or not the insurance is worth it to you. It really is the only question.

Do Mammograms Cause Cancer?

No studies have ever shown that exposure to the small dose of radiation you receive from a mammogram (4mGy) causes cancer. Radiation is known to cause cancer at high doses, but no one knows if it has that capability at such low doses. The risk, if it exists, is so small it has never been observed.

The best evidence available comes from women who were exposed to doses hundreds of times higher than that of a mammogram, such as Japanese women who survived the atomic bomb explosions at Hiroshima and Nagasaki.[19] Based on the number of excess breast cancers in this population, and their estimated radiation dose, mathematical formulas are used to estimate what the cancer-causing potential of a mammogram might be.

The numbers vary with age, but if you are 60 years old, your risk of having a breast cancer caused by a mammogram is roughly 1 in 100,000.[20] Most feel the small risk is far outweighed by the potential benefits of diagnosing the hundreds of naturally-occurring cases at this age at an earlier, more treatable stage.

Keep in mind the risk of radiation-induced cancer from a mammogram is theoretical. No one knows at such low doses if it actually exists. In the interest of radiation safety, the models of potential risk always use worst-case scenarios, which may or may not reflect reality.

Atomic bomb survivors who received up to 250 times the amount of radiation exposure from a mammogram had *no* excess cancers in any group over the age of twenty.[21] The adolescent breast is very sensitive to radiation. The adult breast is surprisingly resistant. The radiation risk models are based on women who received *more* than 250 times the dose of a standard mammogram.

Many experts feel that the effect of periodic exposure to low doses of radiation is not the same as being exposed to a large dose all at once. Tissue damage occurs with each exposure but it's minimal, and because the exposure is periodic, there's plenty of time for the damage to be repaired. This is borne out by animal studies.[22]

Many also believe there is a threshold below which the radiation dose is so small that it has no cancer-causing capability at all. No human studies have been done to confirm this because with doses so small it would have to include tens of millions of women to yield statistically significant results.[23]

As with everything, a little perspective is helpful. We are exposed to background radiation all the time. A mammogram is roughly equivalent to two months background exposure, depending on where you live.[24] This means that two months from now you will have absorbed the equivalent dose of a mammogram from naturally occurring terrestrial and cosmic radiation—just by being alive on planet earth.

The point is, nobody really knows what the radiation risk is from mammography. The risk estimates that are available are derived from mathematical formulas based on dozens of assumptions, which may or may not be true. As nearly as it can be determined, the risk is extremely low, if it exists at all.

As with everything, you have to weigh the potential risks and balance them with the potential benefits. The risk-benefit ratio of mammography seems to come down greatly on the benefit side. Medical X-rays should never be treated casually, but neither should they be avoided like the plague. Mammography is far more likely to save your life than it is to hurt you.

Abnormal Mammograms

The controversy and conflicting information surrounding screening mammography is a little disconcerting, but not overly so, since most women will never get breast cancer anyway. But when you get an abnormal mammogram result, everything changes. Until now, the possibility of breast cancer has been theoretical. But when you get an abnormal mammogram result and realize it really could be you, panic can set in very quickly. As always, having some basic information will be helpful.

The first thing to understand about an abnormal mammogram result is that it isn't necessarily abnormal. It just means you are being called back for extra views to clear up questionable findings on your screening mammogram. This is called a diagnostic mammogram, which is a mammogram done for a symptom such as pain, or a lump, or for questionable screening findings.

The female breast is one of the most difficult organs in the body to image. No other organ varies so much in size and radiographic appearance. In addition, the female breast is a mobile organ attached to the outside of the body, as opposed to the abdominal organs, which are relatively fixed in position.

Because it's soft and pliable, we can't even get meaningful images without compression. Because of this, the radiographic appearance of the breast can vary, not only from year to year, but on different images taken on the same day.

These slight variations in the appearance of the normal breast are usually easy to recognize for an experienced radiologist. But sometimes it can be impossible to tell from a screening examination whether a finding is due to this normal variation or to a small cancer.

Usually one or two extra mammographic views or a breast ultrasound will easily solve this problem. The patient is called and asked to come back for these extra views. The overwhelming majority of cases that are called back are due to these ambiguities rather than a well-defined "abnormality." If you are called back for a diagnostic mammogram because of a finding on your screening mammogram, consider it a "callback" rather than an abnormal result. You will be right more often than not, and save yourself some worry along the way.

Excluding Cancer

Once we've identified those women who can safely return to yearly screening, the remainder must undergo further testing to exclude the possibility of cancer. There are two ways to prove a mammographic finding benign depending on the radiologist's level of suspicion. One is a six-month follow-up, and the other is a biopsy.

A six-month follow-up may sound shocking at first blush. "*What*?" You think I might have cancer, but you're just going to leave it alone for six months? Are you *crazy*?" It may sound like we are. But there is a method to our madness. If your radiologist determines that there is less than a two percent chance that an abnormality is malignant, he or she will recommend you go into the six-month follow-up, or "probably benign" category rather than have a biopsy. This is the standard of care.

This means if we were to biopsy 100 similar abnormalities, we would be performing 98 benign biopsies to find only two cancers. The two cases out of a hundred that do turn out to be cancers are usually small, and very early, typically changing in size by only a few millimeters in the six-month waiting period. They are virtually always the same stage they were six months ago, so literally nothing has been lost.

Remember, only "probably benign" findings are followed. Anything with aggressive features is biopsied. Remember also that you're the one driving the process. If you are uncomfortable waiting, request a biopsy. You won't be upsetting anyone. It happens all the time.

If You Need a Biopsy

Breast biopsies are performed because breast cancer can mimic benign entities on mammography. Breast cancer wears many masks. A biopsy is simply looking behind the mask. We can reliably exclude cancer the vast majority of the time by the mammographic pattern alone, but sometimes things just aren't that clear, and a "tissue diagnosis" is needed. This is nearly always done by a needle biopsy, which is a vast improvement over the days when everyone went to surgery. Today, surgery is largely reserved for women with a breast cancer diagnosis or a questionable finding on a needle biopsy.

Biopsies are rarely performed the same day as the mammogram. They have to be scheduled, usually a few days or a week in advance. Radiologists use either mammographic, sonographic, or MRI images to guide them to the abnormal area, and remove a small piece of tissue through a needle. The tissue is then sent off to a pathologist, who is a doctor trained to recognize disease by looking at cells under a microscope. It is the pathologist who makes the final diagnosis. You are notified of the results usually a day or two after the biopsy.

Women in the middle of the biopsy process almost all say the same thing: the waiting's the worst part. The waiting—and the not knowing. There is some apprehension about the biopsy itself, but the most difficult part is waiting for results after the biopsy. There's something about knowing the next phone call could change your life forever that rocks you to the core.

Since the biopsy process is mostly a waiting game, how well you handle it is about managing your fears while you wait. You can decrease the uncertainty involved by gathering a little basic information at the beginning. You can't get rid of it entirely, but you can decrease the size of the field your fears have to play on. The more you know, the less room your fears will have to run wild.

Find out your radiologist's level of suspicion. He or she should be willing to discuss this with to you, as well as show your mammogram images if it's appropriate. It helps very much to have some idea of what you're dealing with. There's a big difference between a large mass that may well be a cancer, and a tiny area of calcifications that will likely be benign. For the overwhelming majority of biopsies the latter is the case. It helps to know that the odds are in your favor. For every 1000 women screened:[25]

- 80-100 will be called back for extra views or an ultrasound*
- 45-65 of those will have nothing of concern on extra views
- 20 may be asked to return in six months just to be careful
- 15 will be recommended for biopsy
- 2-5 will be found to have cancer

While you're waiting, live your life as normally as you can. Go to work, fulfill your obligations, do whatever you normally do. Focusing on everyday life can be a big help in keeping minor worries in the background. It's natural for your fears to call to you, but as long as they are only a few hecklers in the stands, you can ignore

---

*with the recent FDA approval of 3-D mammography, also called "tomosynthesis," the callback rate is expected to be cut in half. 3-D mammography is available at some women's centers, but it will take several years before its use is widespread.

them and "play your game" like you usually do. It's only when the hecklers leave the stands, come out onto the field, and get in your face that you'll need a different strategy.

When your fears become so strong that they interfere with everyday life, take a break from everyday life. If there's nothing to do, then don't do anything, least of all think. Take a mental vacation. Don't make any important decisions. Don't have any serious discussions with your spouse. As much as possible, put things on hold. Ask those close to you to take up the slack. It would be unusual for them not to step up to the plate, and be happy to do it.

Live in the present moment as much as possible. Understand that you're fighting your negative expectations about the procedure and the possible results—both future events. You aren't fighting "right now," because nothing's happening right now. Your worries are about the future. If you allow yourself to drift off into it, your fears will punish you. So stay anchored in the present moment. It is a safe haven.

Don't go it alone. Share what you're going through with somebody. You don't have to tell everybody about it, but tell somebody. Don't deprive those around you. They love you. If you're not telling them because you're afraid they'll worry—tell them and let them worry. These situations can bring relationships closer together. Like any difficult situation, it's an opportunity. Don't waste it by bearing the entire burden yourself. If you do choose not to share it with anyone, at least keep a journal. It will help dissipate the emotional energy that will surely build if you keep everything to yourself.

If you pray—pray. If you don't—think about starting. At the very least it will keep you focused on the bigger picture. This alone will calm you down. And who knows what else it might do? I've seen more than a few cases where the abnormality had disappeared by biopsy day. There was a rational explanation for most of them.

Chapter Fourteen

For some there wasn't.

As much as possible, **don't let your worries get the best of you.** It's hard to quiet them entirely, but do your best to keep the wolves at bay. Use your waiting time to practice all the stress-reduction techniques we've discussed. If you've been practicing them all along, they'll be readily available. If you haven't, start now.

"Should I worry?" is the number one question I am asked when I'm explaining the need for a biopsy. If the level of suspicion is low, my response is always this: "Though I can't promise you, the chances are this will be benign. If it is, whatever time you spend worrying between now and when you get your results will have been wasted."

Some pre-biopsy concern and apprehension is normal, and probably even healthy. It's good to step back once in a while and take stock of where you are in life. It gives you a chance to make changes you won't make when you're cruising through life on auto-pilot. It's when concern and apprehension turn into worry that you get into problems.

Worry is a form of fear. Nothing good ever comes of it. It's physiologically damaging and it degrades our experience of life. Jerrol Kimmel, R.N., M.A., an integrative health practitioner and faculty member of the Center for Mind-Body Medicine, exposes worry for what it is with her tongue-in-cheek instructions on how to do it: "Go into the future, make something up, and scare yourself today."

It sounds like a ridiculous thing to do when she says it. It seems much more reasonable in the privacy of our own minds. This is a hallmark of our fears. They lose power when they see the light of day; they gain power every time they bounce off a wall in the dark recesses of our mind.

As much as you are able, postpone your worries during the biopsy period. Put them on a shelf and promise you'll get back to them if your biopsy is positive. To take up their concerns now, before you have any concrete information to go on, is of no benefit. Remember, nothing bad has actually happened yet.

Remember also that your biopsy result is something that's beyond your control. Let it be whatever it's going to be, confident that you can deal with what you have to when the time comes. This will help you stay focused on the present and remain at peace. No one expects you to do this perfectly, because we're all human, and we will always be in the process of learning better self-care. None of us will ever master it, so just do the best you can. Consider it a pop quiz on your ability to focus, stay centered, and live in the present moment.

If the Unthinkable Happens

The real craziness begins when you get positive biopsy results. Most women will never see this side of the breast cancer issue, but just under 200,000 a year in the U.S. will. If a benign biopsy is a pop quiz on your ability to stay focused and live in the present moment, a cancer diagnosis is a test that lasts a lifetime.

In the next chapter, we will discuss some of the self-care skills necessary to navigate your way through the cancer maze. It's at this point in the discussion that those simply looking for prevention want to sign off. Thinking about cancer treatment options is the last thing a "healthy" woman wants to do. Most cancer-free women "just can't go there."

This is understandable, but I would urge you to stay the course. Remember, this isn't a book about medical therapy; it's a book about self-care. The skills necessary to navigate your way through cancer diagnosis and treatment are skills that have nothing to do with cancer. They can be applied anywhere.

The things we will learn in the next chapter: how to deal with

Chapter Fourteen

sudden psychological shifts, how to make decisions when the stakes are high and there's little information to go on, and how to remain calm in the midst of life's uncertainties, are skills we all need. "Cancer-free," "cancer patient," and "cancer survivor" are just a few more labels we use to pretend we're somehow different from one another. We're not.

So those who are cancer-free, please read on. If you read between the lines of the discussions that follow, you'll find countless areas in your life where you can use the skills we'll be talking about. It never was about the cancer; it's about something deeper. ❧

15

Navigating the Sea of Uncertainty

❧

One thing that gets lost in the controversies over cancer risk, prevention, and treatment, is how much of an art medicine really is. They say it's both an art and a science, but it's much more of an art *based* on science. Sir William Osler called medicine "the science of uncertainty and the art of probability." This becomes increasingly disconcerting the farther you go in the breast cancer process.

It's understandable when the experts disagree on issues of risk and prevention. It's disconcerting when they can't make up their minds how often you need a mammogram. It's downright frightening when your doctors disagree about your need for radiation or chemotherapy. Suddenly your mortality is staring you in the face, and in the midst of its icy glare, you have to make decisions based on conflicting information. On the good days it's unsettling. On the bad days it can be paralyzing.

The self-care skills we've talked about throughout the book will help you deal with the paralysis. Cancer raises the stakes of the game and cranks the volume of your fears up to high. Mind-body skills, used regularly, will keep you functioning calmly no matter how high the stakes, and will keep your fears from drowning out everything else.

Chapter Fifteen

If you are diagnosed with cancer, these skills are no longer optional—they're mandatory. And it begins with not looking back. No "What ifs" and no beating yourself up. Focus on what you can do something about, and don't waste any mental energy on the rest of it. Breathe, meditate, and live in the moment. Use your imagination to your advantage. Look inward—and upward.

Even though you have cancer, it's important to remember that prevention remains in play. You can't go back and prevent the cancer, but you still have a great deal of influence on your risk of recurrence and survival. Not absolute control—but a great deal of influence.

Seismic Shifts

The physical challenges of breast cancer, especially in the beginning, are not the main issue. Surgery on the breast isn't nearly the physical challenge abdominal surgery is. It's easier, the recovery is quicker, and it's usually done on an outpatient basis. The main challenges of breast cancer are psychological.

The rapid psychological shifts that take place after a cancer diagnosis are some of the most challenging you will ever face. The paradigm shifts we've talked about throughout the book are difficult enough, but those that involve our self-image are the most difficult of all. They are earthquakes of the soul.

The moment you receive a cancer diagnosis, it's impossible to look at yourself the same way again. Others may look at you differently, but the important thing is how you look at yourself. Suddenly you have to deal with your sexuality, your mortality, your relationships at home, and your relationship with yourself. A cancer diagnosis is a blow to the self-image that doesn't go away.

The discomfort and disorientation you feel after a cancer diagnosis is due to your walls crashing down around you. Everything shifts. Nothing is the same. Even familiar things no longer seem familiar. It feels like you're coming apart, and in a psychological sense, you are. It begins on the day of diagnosis and can last weeks, months, or even longer.

How do you deal with these internal seismic shifts? Mostly by being aware of them, and hanging on. The ship will right itself in time. Your walls will reform in a new place, and you will again come into equilibrium—a new normal.

While you're waiting for this to happen, it's important to be patient and gentle with yourself. Do what you have to do and make the decisions you have to make, but try not to do much otherwise. There is some grieving that naturally takes place because the "old you" is gone forever. Allow yourself time to grieve, trusting that a new and better you is right around the corner.

Radical psychological shifts are typical of the cancer world, but not exclusive to it. They occur any time our self-image is jolted by sudden change. Bankruptcy, loss of a loved one, or even the loss of a job can set the same process in motion. The difference is one of degree and depends on what we are most attached to.

Limiting paradigms are like a house of cards: everything is fine until the wind blows. It's not a problem when we find out meditation isn't what we thought it was, or that imagery is more powerful than we knew, but a sudden shift to our self-image rocks us to the core.

This is where your relationships become a powerful resource. Rely on those around you. They see the world more clearly than you can during this time of internal upheaval. Trust them. Lean on them. You need them now more than ever.

The stress surrounding cancer diagnosis and treatment can tear relationships apart, or it can push them closer together. See that it does the latter. Use this time of psychological upheaval to find new and deeper communication with your partner. But don't stop there.

Chapter Fifteen

Reach out to friends, renew old acquaintances—and make new ones.

Group Support

I cannot emphasize enough how important group support is in the cancer arena. Many couples that have wonderful relationships otherwise are unable to talk about their emotions around this issue. She doesn't want to worry or frighten him; he can't deal with the thought of losing her—and neither one can talk about it.

This is not an emotionally healthy situation, even though your relationship is not in danger. We've discussed at length the health risks of bottling up your emotions. It isn't healthy for anyone, but if you have cancer the stakes are a lot higher. Consider emotional work part of your treatment. From a self-care perspective it's exactly that.

Whether your partner can talk about it or not, you *have* to find an outlet where it's safe to express your feelings. The stakes are too high for you not to. You need to be able to laugh and you need to be able to cry. Sometimes it's too hard to do either at home.

There are plenty of support groups around. If you have breast cancer, you won't have trouble finding one. Find one for couples if you can. Partners of people with cancer have special challenges all their own, with far fewer resources to help them. There is a lot of attention given to the cancer patient, but very little given to their partners.

Even if your partner "can't go there," however, you need to. It doesn't have to be a focus group specifically for cancer. Sometimes it's good to have a general mix of people in the group. It will remind you how interconnected we are, and keep you from getting tunnel vision on your particular problem.

The Center for Mind Body Medicine (CMBM) has an excellent

small group model, ideally suited for healing the emotional trauma that results from cancer diagnosis and treatment. They are similar in concept to Dr. Spiegel's groups in that they provide a safe place to express your emotions, learn meditation, imagery, and other mind-body skills, as well as an opportunity to form meaningful and lasting relationships.

I first met Jim Gordon in one of these groups, and you can get a good feel for what one is like by reading his foreword at the beginning of the book. These groups are a phenomenal opportunity for healing. Every time I facilitate one, I am amazed at the transformation I see, both in the group members *and* myself.

There are certified practitioners across the country affiliated with the Center who lead groups in their local area. A list of these practitioners can be found on the Center's website (www.CMBM. org).

There is no evidence that participating in one of these groups will either prevent cancer or prolong survival because no one's done a formal study. There was a research study on melanoma patients that attended a similar group, which met once a week for six weeks (similar to the CMBM model). People who attended the group were found to have significantly decreased mortality *up to six years later* compared those who didn't.[1]

Regardless of breast cancer, the CMBM model has been proven to decrease post-traumatic stress.[2,3] Your psyche doesn't know whether you've been through cancer treatment, shot at in Iraq, lost everything in the floods of Katrina, or family members in an earthquake in Haiti. It just knows it hurts.

No matter what your circumstance, these kinds of groups are simply a good idea. They fall into the zero risk/potential huge benefit category we discussed earlier. Referring to Dr. Spiegel's groups, a leading cancer expert believes "Every cancer patient should be in a group like this."[4] I would disagree only to say that *everyone* should experience a group like this, cancer or not. They are life-changing.

The Art of Decision Making

Once you've braced yourself for the self-image issues that will arise and taken steps to strengthen your relationships, you will need a reliable way to make decisions in the face of all the uncertainty. This is a skill you must have if you are to have any peace in this troubling process, because the information is almost always conflicting, and no matter which path you take, you are in a sense "rolling the dice."

In his book, *The Breakout Principle,* Herbert Benson describes a reliable, scientific, reproducible method for making these types of decisions. This method will work for any decision, but is especially useful in the cancer process where the volume of information can be overwhelming, controversial, and the stakes so high.

Dr. Benson divides the process into three phases, the first of which he calls the **struggle phase**. This might also be called the information-gathering phase. It is strictly an analytical process, based on reason and logic. You gather as much information as you can and analyze the problem from every possible angle, looking for what makes sense and what doesn't. This is the way most of us make every decision, but in Dr. Benson's process, it is only the first phase.

After you've analyzed all the data, you stop wrestling with the problem; you don't keep pushing until you arrive at a decision. For a time at least, you simply drop it. This is called the **release phase.** The point here is to really let the problem go and do something relaxing or meditative. It doesn't matter what you do as long as it is meditative for you. The point is to invoke the relaxation response. This will get you into the proper state of mind for what comes next.

Navigating the Sea of Uncertainty

The third phase is called the **breakout phase**. Benson calls it a "breakout" because the answer comes as a sudden burst of inspiration, often when you least expect it. This is not a process where you chase the answer down with your intellect. Rather, the answer *comes to you*. It's not like hunting quail. It's more like waiting quietly for a dove to alight on your shoulder. The hunting is more satisfying to our rational minds. The waiting is more reliable.

The answer comes effortlessly, as an inner knowing or a gut feeling. Suddenly, from out of the blue, you know on a deep level what you need to do. You may not be able to explain your sudden insight logically, but as long as you've done your homework in the struggle phase, you can trust it.

The classic example of Benson's three-phase process is the apocryphal, but well-known story of Archimedes, a famous Greek mathematician who lived nearly two thousand years ago. The king had charged Archimedes with finding out whether some silver had been mixed in with the gold in a wreath made for one of the temples.

During Archimedes' time, there was no known way of making that determination without melting down the wreath, which he could not do. Despite intense effort, he was unsuccessful in figuring out a solution. Then suddenly, one day while taking a hot bath, the answer came to him.

Knowing that the buoyancy of silver and gold are different, he realized that if he weighed the crown under water, then compared the number to what it weighed on dry land, he could derive the answer. This had to come to him as a sudden insight, because there was nothing in his knowledge base that could have led him to that conclusion.

As the story goes, he was so excited he forgot to put his clothes on and ran down the street naked, shouting "Eureka!" (Greek for *I have found it*) All three phases of Benson's decision-making process can be clearly seen in Archimedes' story, from the struggle phase in his laboratory, to the relaxation phase in the bath, to the breakout phase—his sudden insight.

Benson emphasizes that none of these phases can be skipped. The running down the street naked is optional, of course, but you can't leave out any of the rest of it. The struggle phase primes the pump, but the release phase is just as important. If you skip either one, the breakthrough does not reliably occur. Trust me, the letting go will be a lot harder than the information gathering.

Going for a walk in the woods and continuing to stew over the problem is not letting go. Taking a hot bath while you re-analyze all the data is not letting go. If you have a regular meditation practice, you will know how to let go. If not, this part of the process may be a challenge.

This method makes use of our entire being to make an important decision, not just our analytical brain. We make too many decisions with our reasoning, analytical left brain while completely ignoring our creative, intuitive right brain. We trust far too much in our intellect and far too little in our gut feelings. Both are necessary.

Much of the stress in the cancer journey (and life in general) comes from trying to make decisions from the struggle phase only. This is never a good idea. There's too much information, and too much of it contradictory. Sometimes even what we "know for sure" turns out later not to be true. Trying to make a decision from the facts alone is guaranteed to drive you crazy.

To navigate your way successfully through the cancer maze, remember that information gathering is just that—information gathering. The real decision must come from a deeper place, as reflected in Oriah Mountain Dreamer's advice to a friend with terminal cancer, quoted from her book, *The Call:*[5]

Navigating the Sea of Uncertainty

I can't tell you what to do, because I don't know what you should do...But I have incredible faith in your ability to know for yourself what you need to do...If you can sit with the not knowing, with the fear and confusion and uncertainty that it raises...[and] just simply be still...you will know...what is the best choice for you in this moment...if you can take the time you need to find the deep stillness within, and make your choice from that deep stillness, you cannot make the wrong choice....

As Dreamer's words indicate, you should have a deep peace about whatever decision you come to, whether it's to accept aggressive therapy with possible side effects, or to turn it down. You may not even be able to explain your decision, but you don't have to. You only need to know in your heart it's the right one for you. This inner knowing is what Thomas à Kempis described in his fifteenth-century work, *The Imitation of Christ,* as "What the truth saith inwardly without noise of words."

You will need this deep knowing as time passes because you will be tempted to second-guess yourself all along the way. When you can stand firm in what you know is right for you, despite well-meaning advice to the contrary, you will know you have made the correct decision. It may not be right for anybody else, but it will be for you.

Both Benson's process and Dreamer's advice will help you avoid another common mistake of the cancer journey—making decisions out of fear. The quality of any decision you make depends more on the state of mind you were in when you made it than it does with the details of the decision itself. Inner peace creates a physiologic foundation upon which wise decisions can be made. Fear does the opposite.

A decision-making process that is effective in the midst of any circumstance is (with apologies to Archimedes) worth its weight in gold. We've covered many controversies in this book, but there are many more I couldn't cover. What about thermography? Does Vitamin D prevent breast cancer? What about soy? Does hormone replacement therapy (HRT) affect breast cancer risk?

Many of these will be discussed on my website, www.your-journeytohope.com, as periodic updates. But no matter how many issues I weigh in on, there will always be more. Benson's process will allow you to feel confident making decisions about any of them, even if you are completely on your own.

Perhaps its greatest value is in making what I call the "between-a-rock-and-a-hard-place" decisions so typical of cancer treatment, when every decision is potentially life altering, and must be made in a sea of conflicting information. Should you take chemotherapy or not? On a strictly intellectual level it can be impossible to know. This is perhaps best illustrated by the story of Bonnie, a dear friend Lana and I have known for many years.

Bonnie's Story

We were shocked to hear that Bonnie had been diagnosed with breast cancer. No matter how much you know about the subject, you never think it will *really* be you or someone you love. Bonnie, an attractive woman then in her late fifties, had always been the picture of health. She was active, had a healthy diet, and a positive outlook on life.

Because of the type and size of her tumor when it was discovered, she underwent chemotherapy to shrink it down to a size that would make surgery easier. She responded well to the chemo, and the follow-up surgery was a success. A lymph node sampled at the time of surgery was negative, and she was given a clean bill of health.

Needless to say it was a heavy blow when she received a follow-up phone call after surgery telling her that a second look at the lymph node had revealed cancer cells. In her search for what to do next, she was told by one oncologist that further chemotherapy would be necessary. Another oncologist concurred. Her original oncologist, however, did not agree, saying that she had received all the chemo she needed, and more was unnecessary.

To be on the safe side, she decided to go ahead with the additional chemo, which consisted of 12 separate treatments. After 7 treatments she developed a peripheral neuropathy (numbness of the hands), a known side effect of the chemo. Her doctor told her that if she took further treatments, the numbness could progress and might even be irreversible.

When she asked how it would affect her chances if she stopped after 7 treatments, she was told that nobody knew. There were statistics for women who completed the full course of chemo, and statistics for women who didn't take it at all, but none for women who stopped in the middle.

When she asked about the likelihood of further numbness if she took additional treatments, she was told that it was something no one could predict. It might turn into severe, irreversible numbness, or not progress at all. Every case was different.

So what should she do? If she took further treatments she put herself at risk for potentially life-altering complications, and if she quit she might be placing her life in jeopardy. Her oncologist couldn't help her with the decision since there was no clear answer from a scientific standpoint. And her other oncologist had told her she didn't need the additional chemo in the first place.

What *did* she do? She stopped the chemo, and is doing quite well three years later, learning many of the mind-body skills we've discussed. What would *you* do? You can't know unless you're in that situation. It might be something entirely different—that would be just as right for you as Bonnie's decision was for her.

Chapter Fifteen

Benson's decision-making process is perfect for situations just like Bonnie's, where there is no clear or easy answer. These situations abound in the cancer world, just as they do in life. If we use the peace in our heart as the final arbiter, instead of the accountant in our head, we can be confident of our decision—no matter how little information we have to go on.

A Pitfall

The information-gathering phase begins as soon as you get a diagnosis. With breast cancer, much of it is usually good news. Only twenty percent of those diagnosed with breast cancer will ever die of it. If you've been getting yearly mammograms, the odds are even less it will be you.

Information gathering is easy in the sense that the information you need is the same information you would naturally be curious about: the size of your tumor, how aggressive it is, survival statistics, and so on. Just keep asking questions. The answers will find their way to you.

One pitfall you can run into during your information gathering is especially important. It can come into play at any time, but is common as you consider the possibility of radiation or chemotherapy. It's called relative risk, and it's something to watch out for. The following real-life scenario will illustrate.

After a tumor is completely excised at surgery, radiation therapy is commonly offered as a way of decreasing your risk of recurrence. If you are told the radiation will decrease your risk of recurrence by 50 percent, you might lean toward accepting the therapy, since it sounds like a large benefit. Some small tumors, however, have a recurrence rate of only 6 percent after surgery alone. If you add radiation therapy in these cases the recurrence rate drops to 3 percent.

Navigating the Sea of Uncertainty

Technically speaking, this is a 50 percent reduction. But if only 6 cases out of 100 were going to recur, it means that 94 people would never have a recurrence of their cancer even without the radiation. Additionally, 3 cases out of 100 will recur even with the radiation.

In real numbers, this means that 97 people will be radiated with no benefit at all, and that only 3 will have a recurrence prevented. The actual benefit of radiation therapy in this case is 3 percent, not 50 percent. Additionally, recurrence rate is not the same as mortality rate. Almost no one dies of these small tumors even if they do recur.

This is important to remember because if the information is presented one way (50 percent reduction in risk), you might lean toward accepting radiation therapy, and if it is presented differently (3 percent benefit), you might turn it down.

Relative risk is a comparison of risks between two different groups. Your *absolute risk* is what you need to know. In our example there is a 6 percent absolute risk of recurrence without radiation therapy, and a 3 percent absolute risk of recurrence with it. Yes, one number is 50 percent less than the other, but this has little bearing on the decision you have to make. It is important to remember that *relative risk tells you nothing about your actual risk*. It's only a comparison. Without knowing the risk of both groups being compared, a relative risk value is meaningless.

The same issue presents itself in chemoprevention. The numbers for Tamoxifen use are strikingly similar to our radiation therapy discussion. In the original trial, the cancer rate in the Tamoxifen group was 50 percent less than the control group.[6] But the cancer rate in the control group was only 6 per year per 1000 women, and the cancer rate in the Tamoxifen group was 3 per year per 1000 women.

Again—it *is* a 50 percent reduction. But it also means that 997 women per year took Tamoxifen with no benefit at all, while only

3 cancers were prevented. In another parallel, no decrease in mortality was shown in the Tamoxifen group. Tamoxifen will slightly decrease your risk, but it won't save your life.

Considering the serious side effects of Tamoxifen, which include an increased risk of endometrial cancer, pulmonary emboli, and stroke, you might think differently about taking it depending on how the numbers are presented.

This is not to advise against taking Tamoxifen or radiation therapy. Accepting these treatments will make sense to some women, and not to others. Whether it makes sense to you will depend on how high your risk is, your willingness to tolerate the risk of the side effects, and your overall state of mind. My point is simply that you should find out the real risks and compare them to the real benefits before you decide. Don't just accept a relative number, because it's not the whole story.

Relative numbers can be just as misleading in assessing breast cancer risk factors, though the stakes aren't as high as with treatment options. The 11 percent increase in risk from having one drink of alcohol per day is a good example. Going back to the age-related risk table on page 8, we see that if you are forty years old, your risk of developing breast cancer sometime in the next ten years is 1 in 42.

An 11 percent increase would put your risk at roughly 1 in 38—not a huge difference. It's something you might think about, but not something you're going to lose sleep over. How would it affect your risk if you have a glass of wine with dinner once or twice a week? Nobody knows. That wasn't one of the questions the study asked.

Extrapolating from the one-drink-a-day data, it might increase your risk by 2 or 3 percent. But it might not increase your risk at all. The point is, whether it's for assessing risk factors, evaluating treatment options, or anything in between, relying on relative numbers alone can cause you to wildly overestimate or underestimate your risk. Neither is helpful.

The misleading nature of relative risk is something we face in everyday life, not just in the medical world. Sometimes it's a case of deliberate spin, common in the advertising world. More often it's a case of people knowing just enough about statistics to get them into trouble. Regardless of where you run into it, watch out for relative risk. It's a hole big enough to fall into.

Assess Your True Risk of Breast Cancer, by Patricia T. Kelly, Ph.D., is a great resource if you are presently dealing with the Tamoxifen question or any of the treatment dilemmas involved in the breast cancer journey. There are thorough, down-to-earth discussions of each of these, with all the numbers you'll need.

You *have* to know these numbers to make an informed decision, because for any treatment, there is a degree of risk involved if you accept the treatment, and a degree of risk if you don't. Only you can know which risks you are willing to take; your doctor can't know it for you.

What Grows in Your Garden?

From beginning to end, the uncertainties of the breast cancer issue mirror the deeper uncertainties of life. "Why did this happen to me? Am I going to die? What happens after that? Is there a higher plan, and if so, what's my part in it?" These are the unspoken questions lying just beneath the surface every step of the way. Once you've gotten in touch with them, you've gotten to the real issue, regardless of what's going on with your health.

These questions are unanswerable by our intellect alone. If there is a divine intelligence that pervades the universe and everything in it, we must come to terms with the fact that we will never fully comprehend it. With our intellectual, reasoning minds, it is ultimately unknowable.

With our hearts, however, it's a different story. Ultimately, we can *only* know God with our hearts. Unlike our reasoning minds, our hearts have no problem with the mystery. It's a language the heart intuitively understands.

Our desire for certainty in order to feel safe is a consequence of living life in our heads and closing off our hearts. This is the great disease of Western culture—far more than any physical malady. It's quite likely the *cause* of some of our physical maladies. The Age of Reason has resulted in amazing scientific advances, but caused a disconnect with the deepest part of ourselves.

Requiring absolute certainty before we can be at peace is a quixotic quest, dooming us to forever jousting with windmills. We think if we can "achieve victory" by driving uncertainty into submission this will give us what we want. But what we really want is a deeper connection to God, others, and ourselves. The deepest level of self-care—and the secret of life—is knowing we can never fully have one without the other two.

From a strictly material perspective, the uncertainties of life make no sense, which is why our rational minds make their incessant but exhausting attempts to stamp them out. But from a larger perspective, they make perfect sense—it's impossible to have faith without them. Faith requires unanswered questions or it loses its meaning altogether. Uncertainty, as it turns out, is the only garden faith can grow in. Unfortunately, fear grows in the same garden. Wherever there are roses, there are also thorns.

Thus, the uncertainties of life are both an invitation and a temptation. They invite us to trust in the ultimate goodness of God, and they tempt us to shut down in fear. Can we be at peace in our unknowing, trusting in a higher plan even though we do not understand it? Or will we scramble around on the material plane trying to control everything and everybody around us so we will feel safe?

Faith understands that there is something deeper to this human journey. Deeper even than whether we live or die. Fear understands no such thing. It demands to be in control no matter what. Most of us waffle back and forth between the two, which explains why our experience of life is what it is.

Life is and always will be fundamentally a mystery. Safety and security do not exist on the material plane. They must be found on a higher plane, or they won't be found at all. No matter how much we try to manipulate life, we have no idea what tomorrow will bring. No matter what decisions we make, we can never be sure of the outcome. There can be no guarantees—ever.

Our deepest struggles with the breast cancer issue lead to the same conclusion as so many of life's other struggles—when we leave our spiritual nature out of the equation, it's impossible to solve the equation. ❧

16

I Don't Want to Die

❦

Of all the uncertainties of life, death is the greatest. If awaiting biopsy results feels like canoeing down a river full of alligators, then contemplating our own death is like going over Niagara Falls in a barrel. Death is the great divide. It's the veil that keeps the "other side" shrouded in mystery. If we can come to terms with *that* mystery, we can deal with life's smaller uncertainties more effectively.

At the end of the day, this is what the breast cancer issue comes down to—we don't want to die. After all the layers are peeled away, from the anxiety of mammogram day, to the fearful time awaiting biopsy results, to the terror surrounding cancer treatment decisions, this is what it's about. The breast cancer question brings us face to face with our own mortality. It forces us, briefly for some, more insistently for others, to look in the mirror and see ourselves for what we are: fragile, limited, impermanent.

As frightening as the specter of breast cancer can be, however, it offers an opportunity. It's a chance to awaken. To see life for the gift it really is. To recognize how fleeting and fragile our lives are, understand our place in the universe, and deepen our connection with God. And yet, when we look in the mirror that shows us our mortality, it makes us uncomfortable, and we turn away.

Chapter Sixteen

Most women will never get breast cancer, most of those who do will never die of it, and most who die of it will have years or even decades before death actually comes. Thus, the fear in terms of breast cancer is usually fear of an event—death—that isn't a present reality. For the most part, breast cancer brings us face to face with the *fear* of death, and not death itself. It is an important distinction to make.

Fear is fear. What it attaches itself to is of no consequence. Fear of death is fundamentally no different than fear of flying, fear of snakes, or fear of little red roosters except for a matter of degree. The distinction between death and the fear of death is critical if we're to make any headway in dealing with our emotions surrounding the subject. We won't get far if we think we're dealing with apples but we're really dealing with oranges.

If we look into the face of death and don't like what we see, it's only because we're looking through the eyes of fear. Once our vision improves, we'll see things a lot better. Dealing with fear then, is about learning how to see clearly. It's like cleaning our windshield so we can see the how the world really is. The view is a lot more encouraging than we think.

Understanding Fear

Before we learn how to deal with fear, we first have to understand what it is. Real fear is not something negative. It is tremendously positive. It's part of our nature, given to us as a protective mechanism. Consider Gerald May's experience while he was asleep one night in his tent, as described in his book, *The Wisdom of Wilderness:*[1]

> I sleep again, dreaming…and then a growling that awakens me…I am certain that the growl has come from a close wild presence that is just a few inches from me, just on the…other side…of the

tent…I am terrified and yet I feel a strange calmness…so difficult to describe. It's like some kind of fierce embrace. I lie absolutely still, staring wide-eyed at nothing…My mind appears, thinking fast. What do you do to get rid of a bear?…Nothing to do…"Be frightened. Just be frightened." Nothing to do…The bear paws at something, ambles toward the picnic table…And leaves. Just like that…No more growls. Nothing….My heart is beating so loudly I'm sure the bear hears it. And I have never felt so alive.

For the first time in my life, I am experiencing pure fear. I am completely present in it…there is nothing to do. I have never before experienced such…purity of emotion. This fear is naked. It consists, in these slowly passing moments, of my heart pounding, my breath rushing yet fully silent, my body ready for anything, my mind absolutely empty, open, waiting. I *am* fear. It is beautiful.

What May describes is the pure emotion of fear, what some call natural fear. The bear was real. The fear was real. Natural fear is not something to avoid; we need it. It is a friend, a protector, a preserver of life. As May so eloquently put it, "It's beautiful." If natural fear didn't exist, we'd be playing hopscotch on the highway, walking off cliffs, and trying to swim the Atlantic. Without fear, we'd be a danger to ourselves and everyone around us. Natural fear is a gift. It's part of the software that comes with the human program.

Recalling our earlier discussion on stress, it's easy to pick out the physiological signs of the stress response in May's account: heart pounding, rapid breathing, mental clarity, heightened awareness, readiness for action if it's needed, or stillness if no action is required. In short, readiness to respond in an instant to whatever is called for to improve our chances of survival—in this case, nothing.

It would be easy if that's all there was to it. We could respond appropriately whenever fear strikes us, and move on. The problem comes when we realize there are two distinct kinds of fear—natural fear, and false fear. Some have called it counterfeit fear. The Bible calls it the "spirit of fear." There's an interesting verse on the subject found in the New Testament that gives us some insight into the nature of false fear: *For God has not given us a spirit of fear, but of power and love and of a sound mind.* (2 Timothy 1:7 NKJV)

The first thing this verse tells us is that love and fear are mutually exclusive. The same heart cannot hold both at the same time. One expands our heart and connects us to others. The other contracts our heart and separates us from others. It's been said that every action we take in life is taken either out of love or out of fear.

It's also clear that we give our power away when we accept false fear as real. This is yet another example of the power of faith. When we invest it in our fears, they become reality to us. Believing an illusion is just one more way we give our power away.

We just as clearly forfeit a sound mind when we accept a false fear as the truth. This also makes sense from a physiologic perspective. It's just one more reason not to make any decisions out of fear. Our physiology guarantees they won't be good ones.

The following are some characteristics that can help us differentiate between the two types of fear. Realize that we will experience the same emotional response and the same physiologic response for either of them. Both will *seem* real to our minds, and both will *be* real to our bodies.

Real Fear	False Fear
Expands awareness	Diminishes awareness
Based on truth	Based on illusion
Alerts us to present danger	Concerns a possible future danger

I Don't Want to Die

Dealing with fear is the same as dealing with any other emotion. It begins by being aware of what we're feeling. If we can manage not to deny our fear or repress it, it's only a matter of figuring out if it's real or not. The table above gives us several ways to go about it.

It's difficult to judge our level of awareness. Our awareness varies from moment to moment, and we can only be as aware as we are at any given time. From our perspective, our awareness level is always 100 percent of whatever it is. It always seems the same to us, even though others can notice the difference quite easily.

It can also be difficult to tell the difference between what's real and what's not. That's obvious by how successful illusions can be. Lies would never work if they didn't resemble the truth. A wolf in sheep's clothing will fool us sometimes, but a wolf that comes as a wolf never will. An illusion that's obvious isn't an illusion. All our fears seem real even if they're not, so reality is no more useful than judging our level of awareness.

This leaves us with the easiest, quickest, and most obvious way to tell the difference between real and false fear, which is to determine whether the "problem" is something that's happening right now, or only a future possibility. Real fear is the fear of real death, this moment, right now. Anything else is a counterfeit.

When you receive the news of an abnormal mammogram, or the need for a biopsy arises, it's easy to rush off into fearful thoughts about having cancer, followed by radiation and/or chemotherapy and the possibility of dying. Though these are a distinct possibility for some, they have nothing to do with the present moment.

The fearful mind can be off to the races long before the rational mind can catch it. The trick is to build your self-awareness through meditative practice so you can catch the stress response before it's too late to rein it in. It's also helpful to have tools such as simple breathing techniques available to anchor your mind and calm yourself down.

When fear strikes, simply ask yourself, "Is there a problem *right now?*" It's a simple question, but in terms of fear it will cut to the chase immediately. If there is an immediate problem, then deal with it. But if you even have time to ask the question, you're probably dealing with false fear. When bears actually do show up, we usually run first and ask questions later, May's case being a rare exception.

False fear has been described by the acronym F.E.A.R., which stands for *false expectations appearing real.* Fear is an expectation, no more than a guess about what the future might hold. The thing we fear *might* happen, but it might not.

Counterfeit fear tricks us into survival mode when no present problem exists. We say things we shouldn't say and do things we shouldn't do under its influence. The trick is not to be "under the influence." The easiest, most reliable way to do that is to live in the present moment as much as possible.

Just asking yourself the question, "Is there a problem right now, in this moment?" is a powerful antidote to fear because it brings you back to the present, where false fear cannot exist. Get used to asking this of yourself. And if you don't get a clear answer, then that's your answer.

It's been said that all fear is some variation of the fear of death. The reality of death is something we all acknowledge intellectually, but few of us have contemplated deeply. We ignore the subject because it frightens us.

For those in touch with ultimate reality, death is considered more of a graduation. This friendly relationship with death is not just the birthright of a few enlightened souls, however. It can be that way for all of us if we're willing to do the work. And the work is dealing with our fears around the subject.

I Don't Want to Die

What Are We So Afraid Of?

No culture on the face of the earth is as disconnected with death as ours. Not many of us have ever seen a dead body. We mostly send our elderly somewhere else to die, not at home. In hospitals, we immediately cover dead bodies with a sheet because seeing one makes us uncomfortable.

To see a dead body is, in a sense, to look upon our own mortality—and mostly we don't like what we see. In our culture, we are so identified with material forms that the mere thought of losing these forms evokes intense fear. If we believe this physical form is who we are, then we greatly fear its dissolution. Well-known Buddhist monk, Thich Nhat Hanh, puts it this way in his book, *No Death, No Fear:*[2]

> Our greatest fear is that when we die we will become nothing. We believe that we are born from nothing and that when we die we become nothing. And so we are filled with the fear of annihilation.

But death doesn't mean we become nothing. We never were nothing, and we never will be. Our fear of death betrays our material view of life. We assimilate many of our beliefs from our parents, but we also absorb the beliefs of the culture into which we are born. In our case, that culture is a strongly material one. We say we are "spiritual beings having a human experience," but our fear of death betrays that our deeper beliefs are more akin to Thich Nhat Hanh's analysis.

The phrase, "spiritual beings having a human experience," while true, has lost its power to inspire us due to overuse. It's much like the word "love." Once you hear it enough times, it rings hollow. Let's look at a few metaphors that tell us essentially the same thing.

Chapter Sixteen

Our Essential Nature

Every human being is like a house. The house is made up of four walls, a roof, and the space inside. If the house burns down, we say it ceases to exist, but this is only from a material standpoint. The space inside is completely unaffected. It's the same as it was before, only now it's connected with the space outside of where the four walls once stood. The truth is, it was always connected to the outside. Only our material point of view gave us the illusion that it wasn't. From the point of view of the space, "inside" or "outside" never had any meaning.

The life in a house occurs in the space, not in the physical walls. The walls and the roof are only the container. The life it contains is, was, and always will be connected to everything else. The life has nothing to do with the four walls—and never did.

We can also be likened to a wave in the ocean. A wave has a beginning and an end, but it is always water. When the wave ceases to exist, the water that made it does not cease to exist. Every molecule of water that made up the wave is still somewhere. Each wave has a "birth" and a "death," but the essence of the wave (the water) never ceases to exist.

Hanh also likens our existence to making a pot of oolong tea:

> The tea leaves are placed in a pot, and boiling water poured on them. Five minutes later there is tea to drink. When I drink it, oolong tea is going into me...After I have poured out all the tea, what will be left in the pot is just the spent tea leaves. The leaves that remain are only a very small part of the tea. The tea that goes into me is a much bigger part...It is the richest part. We are the same; our essence has gone into our children, our friends and the entire universe. We have to find ourselves in those directions and not in the spent tea leaves.

I Don't Want to Die

The space within the four walls, the water in the wave, and the essence of the tea all represent our spirit or our True Nature. Our True Nature has no fear because it knows it will go on no matter what. It always has been and it always will be. Fear of dying is a symptom of our forgetfulness more than anything else. In our journey through this material realm, we've forgotten who we really are.

Even from a material viewpoint, our traditional notion of death begins to break down when we look a little closer. On a cellular level, we're dying and being reborn all the time. Each and every cell in our body is pre-programmed for a certain lifespan, which differs with each cell type. Cells in the GI tract live only for a few days, red blood cells for a few months, and bone cells for a few years.

Each cell is programmed for a certain number of cell divisions and then the cell, unable to reproduce further, dies. This pre-programmed cell death is called *apoptosis*. The process of cellular death and rebirth is going on all the time. By the time you finish reading this sentence several million of your cells will have died and been replaced with new ones.

Life and death are intertwined throughout nature. If you look around in a healthy forest, you'll see dead and dying trees everywhere. An old rotten log with flowers and young saplings growing out of it is a common sight in any forest. Death, quite literally, is the breeding ground of new life. And so it is with us. Without the interplay between living and dying cells, life could not exist.

Understanding apoptosis makes it even more obvious that we are not and cannot be only a physical body. As we discussed in an earlier chapter, the ongoing process of cellular renewal assures that roughly every seven years each cell in our body will be replaced. So if your definition of dying is the death of the body, then you have already died! Several times, depending on how old you are.

Chapter Sixteen

Who am I, then? At every age, I've felt like "me." Other than a few aches and pains, I don't feel any different now than I did in all my other physical iterations. And when I die, which "me" is going to heaven: the child, the adolescent, or the mature man? The answer, of course, is that it's the wrong question, because none of these was or is the real me. My body turns over every so often, but my essence does not.

We come to this planet to experience a limited existence, and seem to promptly forget that our essence remains *un*limited. We mistake our earth suit for "us." But we are not the suit; we are the wearer of the suit. We are not the wave; we're the water. We are not the house; we're the life within the house.

If we misunderstand death, it's because we're trying to explain it from a material point of view. The house metaphor makes this clear. When we die, the soul doesn't leave the body, it's the other way around. Our soul doesn't go anywhere because "where" is a strictly material phenomenon. Death is a transition from the material realm to the eternal realm. It is a vehicle, but it doesn't just take us from here to "there." It takes us from here to *everywhere*. Linda Sylvester describes this beautifully in her song, "Bridge To All That Is."*

When we keep our spiritual nature in mind, death is not the clear-cut entity we have always considered it. Conventional medicine looks at death as the enemy, something to be conquered at all costs. But is it really? No spiritual tradition teaches that physical death is the end of the line. They may differ in what it looks like, but every religion has an afterlife in its worldview. Should we really look to a medical system that ignores two-thirds of our mental, physical, and spiritual nature as the final word on the subject?

Of all those who have had near death experiences—where they

*See page 259

briefly die, pass over to the other side, and are then revived—virtually none report wanting to come back. So how bad can it actually be? Consider the comment of Socrates, a character in the movie, *The Peaceful Warrior*: "Death? It's a transformation. A little more radical than puberty, perhaps, but nothing to be afraid of."

Fear of death is the hallmark of the breast cancer journey. Even the other issues involved—loss of sexuality, loss of self-image, and so on, can be seen as variations on the same theme. We'll lose our sexuality completely when we die. Our self-image as it relates to our bodies will be torn away as well, because when we die we'll "lose" that too. What the breast cancer question offers from beginning to end is the opportunity to see this. It whispers it gently once a year on screening mammogram day. It screams it every day to those with advanced cancer.

Keeping this bigger picture in mind helps tremendously in negotiating your way through the breast cancer maze. It isn't really about dying because we're all going to die at some point. Even if you have advanced cancer, it's not about dying; it's about how you choose to live in the face of dying. I can think of no better way to illustrate this than by the following story.

Ron's Story

Ron Kurtz and his son, Randy, built our home in Naples, FL almost 20 years ago. Ron, originally from Iowa, used to tell me how he built houses for people back home on a handshake, with no contract at all. We did have a contract, but I always trusted Ron more than I did the contract. I considered Ron and Randy's word the real thing. And it always was. They built us a beautiful home, where we still live, and as happened with so many of their clients, we became friends.

Chapter Sixteen

Some years later, shortly before Ron's sixtieth birthday, he was diagnosed with advanced colon cancer, and given less than a year to live. None of his doctors wanted to be very aggressive because of his poor prognosis. The situation was grim, to say the least. At the time of his diagnosis, Ron had recently finished building a house for a client who happened to be a major contributor to a cancer center in Ohio.

After a few phone calls, connections were made and Ron flew up for a consult. He was offered hope, but at the price of aggressive surgery and chemotherapy. Ron decided to take the chance, and so began his final odyssey.

To the surprise of most of his doctors, but probably not to Ron and his family, the cancer went into remission and Ron lived another six years. They weren't six carefree years by any means. There were many complications, recurrences, and additional surgeries. In the end, Ron was left with only a few feet of small bowel, which made eating and absorbing fluids a terrific problem. Ron did eventually die from complications of his cancer, but it was long after the one-year sentence had been pronounced. Fifteen hundred people attended Ron's memorial service, a huge number for such a small town.

Shortly before Ron's death, his family had a DVD made of a friend interviewing him about his life. An excerpt from the interview was played on the overhead screen at the memorial service. Ron discussed during the interview what his cancer journey had been like, and his eager anticipation of what came next. His strong Christian faith allowed him to be confident of his future in spite of his impending death. I don't remember many details from the video. I only remember being shocked when he said, "The last six years have been the best years of my life."

"*What!? The best six years of your life? How could that possibly be?"* I wondered to myself. I had been working at the hospital many times when Ron came in due to complications. I would always take a look at his X-rays, and then go spend a few minutes visiting with him. We'd catch up, and I'd let him know what was going on from an insider's perspective.

I saw all the recurrences, and the obstructions, and the many emergency surgeries. Being in the medical field, I knew the physical suffering he experienced. And I'm quite sure I only saw the tip of the iceberg. Only Ron and his family knew how tough it really was. Those six years were not a bed of roses for Ron by any stretch, and yet at the end he said, quite sincerely, that they'd been the best six years of his life. His statement affected me deeply, and still does.

I didn't understand at the time, but it seems clearer looking back at it. Ron had always loved his family. He constantly spoke about how proud he was of them, even before he got sick. After his diagnosis, he had six full years to spend with them when he knew every day might be his last.

How many "I love yous" did Ron leave unsaid in those six years? None, I should think. How much did he appreciate the small things—a few minutes with the grandkids, a quiet conversation with his wife, lunch together with a friend? Immensely, I'm quite sure. He soaked up each moment, taking in every bit of joy there was to be had.

Yes, upon deeper reflection, I understand exactly what Ron was talking about. He eventually succumbed to the cancer, but the cancer never beat him. He lived his last six years moment-to-moment, with an aliveness that most of us who are cancer-free never do. Why not? Because we think we have plenty of time. Ron knew better.

Ron's story embodies so much I want to say about death and dying—and living. Some might question why I would even use the story of a man who died of colon cancer in a book about breast cancer when there are plenty of breast cancer stories to tell.

I use it because it's meaningful on so many levels, and because it still moves me. I tell it because living is living and dying is dying. We separate ourselves in so many ways: by gender, disease, physical appearance, or by the flag that flies over the piece of the earth we happen to call home. Ron's story is our story, no matter who we are, where we're from, or whether we ever have to deal with cancer or not.

Ron is a perfect example of Hanh's oolong tea. I was so taken by his strong faith, love of family, and courage in the face of tremendous physical challenges that his story made its way onto these pages. As I recount it, I can still feel his presence. His essence is part of me and will always remain so. And now it's part of you. Is Ron really gone? On one level of reality, yes. But on another, no—his essence is still here.

Ron is an example of what Bernie Siegel calls an "exceptional cancer patient," one who lives far longer than statistics say they should.[3] If you have cancer, you can take hope from the fact that the world is full of them.

Exceptional Cancer Patients

The goal of most people reading this book is not to be a cancer patient at all. The best way to do that is to emulate what it takes to be an exceptional cancer patient before you actually are one. Rather than labeling them as patients, I prefer to call them exceptional people living with cancer. These exceptional people:

- Don't consider themselves victims
- Focus on their health, not their disease
- Focus on living, not dying
- Maintain strong relationships

- Take an active role in their health
- Are optimistic
- Don't dwell on the past
- Have an active spiritual life
- Maintain a grateful attitude
- Don't complain
- Don't fear death

Exceptional people living with cancer didn't necessarily start out that way. The exceptional ones are those who let their cancer journey mold them into something they may have always wanted to be anyway. The cancer experience is a crucible, there's no doubt about that. Cancer is the potter's wheel in every sense of the word.

Cancer isn't what any of us want, but if you find yourself in the fire, you have two choices: you can kick and scream, in which case the fire will consume you, or you can accept the situation as it is, and allow the fire to make you into a beautiful vessel. If the fire isn't going away, only one choice makes sense.

Not everyone will be cured of cancer, no matter how exceptional they are. If death is a river we all have to cross, cancer is the boat some of us will have to take. Everyone can be *healed* of cancer though, even if they aren't cured. The word "healing" comes from the same root word as "whole" and "holy." It has nothing to do with being cured, which describes an absence of disease.

A cure has to do with the body; healing occurs in the soul. Healing is about being fully integrated with ourselves, not fragmented into different parts headed in different directions. We've visited this concept before in terms of our projections, which makes it clear that healing has nothing to do with whether we live or die.

What does someone look like who is healed? They display most of the attributes in the above list. These don't develop overnight. They unfold to the degree that one surrenders to the process. Every difficulty in life is an opportunity, and cancer is no exception. With the proper perspective, cancer can be a path to healing, wholeness, and spiritual awakening. What is the purpose of life if not this?

Acceptance

It seems paradoxical that those who aren't afraid to die tend to live longer, but it makes sense both energetically and physiologically. Fear is negative imagery. It's the mental equivalent of hanging depressing pictures on your wall and staring at them all day. This makes what you don't want *more* likely, not less.

Fear also causes chronic stress. By brooding over a possible negative future event that we cannot change, we create an unsolvable problem—an inherently stressful situation. If stress is damaging to a healthy body, it's only going to make things worse if you have cancer.

There are three reasons people don't want to die:

1. They're afraid of it
2. They don't want to leave loved ones
3. They feel they have a God-given purpose in life they haven't accomplished yet.

The first two of these are fear-based. The third is not. Interestingly, the majority of spontaneous healings occur in the last group. There's a world of difference between not wanting to die and wanting to live. Even if a miracle is not in the cards for you, accepting the reality of death releases you from your struggle with something you have no control over. Paradoxically, this tends to extend life.

Acceptance, sometimes referred to as surrender, is powerful. Acceptance is not resignation or quitting. It means abandoning the struggle against what is; that we quit demanding something different of life than what it's already given us. When we accept how things are in the present moment, we are brought into alignment with God. And that's a good place to be, whether you're going to spend a little more time here with us, or you're headed into eternity.

Ron accepted his situation, but he never quit. He went out of his way to take more aggressive treatment than many of his doctors recommended. The only time he missed a treatment was to go on trips with friends and family. He lived life fully as long as it was there to be lived, yet was ready to go at any time. This is acceptance.

He mentioned several times in his interview how excited he was to go to heaven. He said there were times when he went to sleep thinking he was going to die, and was a bit disappointed when he woke up to find himself still here. He wanted to stay with his family as long as possible, but he reminded me of a little kid at Christmas when he talked about moving on.

There's a traditional Indian saying: "When you were born, you cried and the world rejoiced. Live your life in such a manner that when you die the world cries and you rejoice." Ron did that—perhaps better than anyone I know.

A Balanced Perspective

A little apprehension concerning death is normal. But there's no reason for terror. It should be more like closing your eyes and jumping out of a tree because your father promised he'd catch you. As you're about to jump, it's normal for some doubt to creep in, and for your heart to leap into your throat as you're falling. But your Father *will* catch you, just like he promised.

It is the reality of death that best teaches us how to live. Ask any soldier what life was like during war. Aside from the fear and horror of combat, he will usually describe an intense sense of aliveness.

Chapter Sixteen

Why? Because a soldier knows each day could be his last. The rest of us live under the illusion that tomorrow is somehow promised to us. It isn't.

Having a healthy perspective on our mortality is the key to a healthy perspective on life. The benefits are enormous. A balanced view of death:

Gives us a proper perspective of time. When we understand how limited our time here really is, we waste a lot less of it. Only when something is limited is it considered valuable. Gold is valuable; lead is not. Each grain of sand in the hourglass is precious; a grain of sand on the beach, nearly worthless.

Transforms our relationships. Sure, it would be a lot easier to get along with your partner if you only had to live with them for the next thirty minutes instead of the next thirty years. But if each moment of the next thirty years you acted as if you only had thirty minutes, your love story would be one they'd write ballads about.

Encourages us to find our life purpose and get busy doing it. When we think we'll be around forever, we don't feel any urgency. When we know we won't, it helps us focus on what's important.

Leads to a life of gratitude. This may be the most important and encompasses the other three. The moment anything comes to us in life, it is already passing away. Nothing on the material plane will last forever—no person, no thing, no situation. When we realize this, it naturally leads us to be grateful for all of it. And a grateful life is a great life, from any perspective. ๛

I Don't Want to Die

Bridge To All That Is

Take my hand and follow me.
Open your eyes, come and see.

There's a secret place for you and me
Across the bridge to all that is.

Meet me at the door to forever.
We'll dance into the bright sunlight.

Share secrets of eternity together.
Watch the world unfold with delight.

And we'll live.
Life will never end.

In all that is.

Just reach out.
Just reach in.
Just let go, and enter in.

There's a whole new world
For you and me
Across the bridge to all that is....

[with permission. Linda Sylvester]
www.LindaSylvesterMusic.com

17

Gratitude

❧

If love is the king of emotions, then gratitude is surely queen. The two are intertwined in a mysterious but unmistakable way. It's impossible to feel love without feeling some degree of gratitude. How much of that wonderful sensation we feel in our chest is love and how much is gratitude is impossible to tell. Consider the words of Gerald May after another terrifying experience in the wild:[1]

> Thank you, God. Oh, God, I thank you. I am flooded by an immense feeling of gratitude. I am filled with it…The thankfulness feeling is overwhelming, so strong I cannot tell it from love. What is this…Terror-life-thanksgiving-love-power. My heart is thrashing from fear inside my chest, breath full, deep, clean, senses pure, vital….And oh, this mind, this awareness. Nothing inside but the clear radiance of living. God, I am so grateful, so overcome with thanksgiving for sheer being…Thank you, thank you, oh, thank you. I could die now, for I know what life is…oh my divine love, never again reassure me. I do not want to know everything will be all right. I never want to be secure again as long as I live. Give me no safety. Only give me this livingness forever….

The indescribable feeling May does his best to describe shows the lack of a clear boundary between love and gratitude. The intense aliveness he felt so grateful for is the expansiveness and interconnectedness we have discussed throughout the book. It comes to us when our boundaries fade, self begins to disappear, and we sense our connectedness to everything in existence.

It is reality knocking. And May quite elegantly describes what we miss when we don't answer the door. This at-oneness moment, a state of awe and wonder when time stands still, is sometimes called gratefulness to distinguish it from merely being thankful for a material possession or a pleasant circumstance.

Gratitude is a spectrum, beginning with **intellectual gratitude**, which consists of brief thankful thoughts for a person, thing, or event. The next step is **heartfelt gratitude**, a physical sensation, usually perceived in the chest, which can be considered an emotion. The highest level is **gratefulness**, the expansive, at-oneness experience May described. As with everything else, it doesn't pay to get too hung up on the words. The ends of the spectrum are clearly different, but as you progress from intellectual gratitude, to heartfelt gratitude, to gratefulness, one blends imperceptibly into the other.

In his book, *Thanks*, Robert Emmons describes gratitude as "a feeling, a moral attribute, a virtue, a mystical experience, and a conscious act, all in one."[2] A French proverb calls gratitude "the memory of the heart." Whatever words you use to describe it, gratitude is something to be coveted. If the full spectrum of gratitude is a five-course meal, you won't want to leave anything on your plate.

What Gratitude Can Do for You

Having a few thankful thoughts here and there may or may not be helpful, depending on how fleeting the thoughts are. Cultivating a consistently grateful attitude, however, will bring you everything you want. If you're willing to take it on as a challenge, and work at it with the same diligence you would if you took up tennis or decided to learn a new language, you'll end up one of the happiest people on the planet.

People with a thankful attitude feel better about their lives, are more optimistic, report fewer physical complaints, and spend more time exercising. Not surprisingly, they show higher levels of alertness and feel more alive. Grateful people are more likely to report having helped someone with a personal problem or offered emotional support to a friend in the recent past.[3] Thus, positive social behavior is a consequence of feelings of gratitude.

Heartfelt gratitude gives you free access to your inner pharmacy. That sweet feeling in your chest lets you know the drug cabinet is wide open. It's like having your own morphine pump to dull the pains of life, with the exception that the side effects help you think *more* clearly, and make you *more* aware of what's going on around you, not less.

Gratitude decreases our perception of physical pain, and increases the strength and coherence of our cardiac field. Heartfelt gratitude gets our energies humming, allowing our bodies to function at their highest level. Gratitude even appears to affect longevity. One study showed that nuns who reflected more gratitude in their journals lived significantly longer than their less thankful counterparts.[4]

A grateful attitude strengthens social bonds and friendships. Among all the emotions, gratitude is the one that, more than any other, accounts for the presence or absence of stress in relationships.[5] That alone makes it something to be coveted. According to Emmons, "When we give the gift of gratitude with the right spirit, genuinely from our heart, we get as much or more in return for giving the thanks as the receiver gets from receiving it."

Happiness can be measured by the amount of gratitude in one's heart. Happiness has been defined as "wanting what you have," but

Chapter Seventeen

"being thankful for what you have" is an equally good definition. Happiness is a perception. It has nothing to do with how things really are. If I perceive myself to be happy, then by definition, I am happy. People who have a consistently grateful attitude are some of the happiest people anywhere.

Gratitude is also an effective counterbalance to our desires. There's nothing wrong with desiring something. It's only when we forget to be thankful for what we already have that it gets to be a problem. The desire for more, without gratitude, can be defined as greed. Wealth is a state of mind, not a number. A grateful attitude gives us the state of mind, no matter what the number is. Greed is a perpetual state of lack no matter how much you have.

Anger, rage, and resentment, much like greed, cannot coexist with gratitude. Our hearts are big enough to hold one or the other, but not both at the same time. Giving gratitude a home in our hearts keeps these "wolves" at bay. And when we occasionally give in to the wolves, allowing gratitude back into our hearts will make them disappear faster than vampires at sunrise.

Gratitude is an upward spiral. The more grateful we are, the more reasons we find to be grateful. The act of gratitude itself raises our awareness of blessings we already have. Thus, gratitude is a meditation in addition to all the other things. The blessings are already there; we only have to notice.

Gratitude not only increases our perception of blessings, it may actually bring us more of them. This has not been scientifically proven, but it's considered self-evident to many. Teachings from every spiritual tradition tell us we'll get more of whatever we are thankful for. If you want to test the Law of Attraction, gratitude is a good place to start.

Gratitude

Gratitude and Spirit

Gratitude is an integral part of every spiritual tradition, across every culture. Praise of God, love of God, and worship of God all have a degree of gratitude contained within them. An attitude of thanksgiving is seen as being the only reasonable stance humans can take toward their Creator.

In a sense, every thank you is a spiritual act. Every thank you, followed to its logical conclusion, is a prayer. Consider the simple case where your arms are full of groceries and a stranger opens the door for you. You say, "Thank you," but who are you thanking? Who taught this man to be so kind? His parents? In a sense then, you're thanking his parents too. But where did they learn it? Aren't you partly thanking their teachers as well?

And he didn't show up randomly just when you needed him. What about those who produced the car that brought him to you? Or the mechanics that keep it running? Or the employer that pays him so he can afford to have it? No matter where you begin or how far you take it, it always ends up at the same place—infinity.

Where did it all start? Where did we come from, and how did we get here? We can thank our "lucky stars," but if we're only here by luck because the stars just happened to align, then no thanks are necessary because there's no one to thank.

Gratitude requires a potential receiver or it has no meaning at all. The mere fact that human gratitude exists is some of the most compelling evidence that there *is* Someone to thank. And the thanks, no matter how they're offered up, are always welcome. Meister Eckhardt, a Christian mystic from the Middle Ages, put it this way, "If the only prayer you ever say in your entire life is 'Thank you,' it will be enough."

All we have to know about the spiritual nature of gratitude may be contained in the word itself. Gratitude is closely related to the word "grace," which means divine favor. Both words are derived from the Latin word *gratus*, which means "thankful, or pleasing," which comes from a much older Sanskrit word, *grnati*, meaning "sings, praises, or announces." In Italian, the words for "thank you," *grazie*, and "grace," *grazia*, are nearly identical. This is how the phrase, "saying grace" before a meal originated. The French word for "thank you" is *merci*, which is related to our word "mercy."

The Eucharist, a term used to describe the Christian sacrament of Communion, is derived from the Greek *eucharisteo*, which means "thanksgiving." *Eucharisteo* in turn is related to the Greek roots *charis*, meaning "divine favor or gift," and *chara*, which means "joy."

Mercy, grace, divine favor, gift, sings, praises, joy. Is there anything else that needs to be said?

Gratitude in Adversity

It's easy to count our blessings when life is going well; it's something else entirely to remain thankful when difficult times hit. Adversity puts gratitude to the test like nothing else. We will all be touched by pain and sorrow at some point in our life. The only question is, how will we deal with them when they come? Sometimes when our hearts break, it's hard to keep the gratitude from leaking out.

The key to weathering tough times is to maintain our perspective. Pain, emotional or physical, draws our focus like a laser beam. But when we allow our attention to be drawn to what's not going well in our lives, it's all too easy to forget about what *is* going well. Maintaining a grateful attitude in adversity is all about remembering. It's not denial in the face of tragedy. It's simply keeping a larger perspective.

If you find yourself indulging in self-pity or complaining, you can be sure gratitude has flown the coop. These narrow our focus so severely it can be embarrassing. If you struggle with back pain, for instance, you won't get much sympathy from those in a wheelchair. If your knee hurts, there are lots of amputees who would love to have your problem. And there are a host of young women who will never live long enough to worry about breast cancer.

Finding the Gift

Maintaining gratitude in the midst of difficult circumstance is not only about remembering our blessings; it's about finding the gift in the new circumstance. There are many levels of reality. What is a tragedy on one level is always a gift on another. Every tragedy presents us with an opportunity, even if it's "only" an opportunity to develop our character.

Ron found the gift in his cancer. He would never have wished for the cancer, but in return for having to struggle with it, he was presented with what he considered an unparalleled gift. On the surface, it would seem that he got a bum deal, but he obviously didn't think so. Given the cards he was dealt, he played his hand spectacularly.

The good news is that we don't have to wait for cancer to find the gift; there is a gift in everything. The New Testament tells us:

...in all things God works for the good of those who love him...
(Romans 8:28 NIV)

Byron Katie states this another way when she says, "Everything happens for me. Nothing happens to me." This attitude shows trust in a higher purpose. It allows us to find the blessings hidden right before our eyes.

Gratitude is not a state in which suffering and adversity are selectively ignored. Rather, gratitude makes us focus on the opportunity adversity offers, the opportunity of authentic spiritual growth. This turns suffering into growing pains. Complaining turns suffering into more suffering.

Most have forgotten that fully half the Pilgrims died their first winter in the New World. Only three families were untouched by the death of a husband, wife, or child.[6] Robert Emmons had this to say about them:

> Their thankfulness was not a selective, positive thinking façade, but rather a deep steadfast trust that goodness ultimately dwells even in the face of uncertainty. Their thanksgiving was grounded in the actuality that true gratitude is a force that arises from the realities of the world, which all too often include heartbreak, sometimes overpowering heartbreak.

Hindrances to Gratitude

All hindrances to gratitude boil down to focusing on the self. When we forget our interconnectedness to and interdependence on others, we fall back into the illusion of separateness. Feeling self-sufficient, we find it difficult to be grateful.

Emmons, perhaps the world's pre-eminent researcher on gratitude, says that he must remind himself a thousand times a day how much he depends on others or he cannot maintain a grateful attitude. No matter what we accomplish in life, we never do it alone. We always stand on someone's shoulders, no matter what the endeavor. No man is an island—ever.

If we think we've accomplished everything on our own, then there's no need to be thankful for it. As Bart Simpson said when Homer asked him to say grace before dinner, "Dear God, we bought all this stuff ourselves, so thanks for nothing!" Though few of us would ever utter these words, Bart's statement embodies what many of us say with our attitudes: "I've earned this, so gratitude isn't necessary—I deserve it."

Taking things for granted is just another way of saying we deserve them. If one feels entitled to everything, then one is thankful for nothing. Complaining is a sign of this sense of entitlement. Complaints are basically demands of life to "do things my way." The fact that life usually isn't impressed with our demands doesn't seem to stop us from making them. If we understood that there's not a shred of gratitude in complaining, we might think twice before doing it.

A feeling of indebtedness is also a sign of an inability to feel gratitude. When we find ourselves saying, "I owe you one," or feeling like we need to return the favor when a simple "thank you" would do, it's a signal that underneath we don't feel worthy of the gift.

One of the biggest obstacles to gratitude is that we just don't take the time. Simply taking the time to count our blessings is one of the best ways to experience the fullness and joy of life. Few of us slow down long enough to make a decent effort at it.

Cultivating Gratitude

Gratitude is a skill that can be developed. It can be acquired by simple practice. There is no gratitude gene that predisposes one to be thankful. Gratitude is something anyone can learn.

If you are serious about cultivating a grateful heart, the first thing to do is make it a firm intention. **Set it as a definite goal.** Make a commitment to yourself that you're really going to do this. I suggest adding it to the list you made in chapter nine if it isn't there already. You will have to replace something if you've already done the exercise, but that's okay. Whatever you choose to replace on your list—this is more important.

Considering the multi-faceted nature of gratitude and its tendency to grow over time, having a grateful attitude may be more important than your whole list. The process of setting a goal, seeing it in your mind's eye, and focusing on it with patience and persistence, will work in any area of your life. Why not use it toward becoming more thankful, which will enhance every area of your life?

Set aside the time. It isn't going to happen unless you practice. The good news is that it's a lot easier to fit in your schedule than you might think. Don't forget, gratitude itself is a meditation, and can fit into whatever meditation practice you already have. Gratitude is also easily incorporated into prayer. Prayers are more powerful when they come from a firm foundation of gratitude. And if you can't pray out of gratitude, you can always pray *for* gratitude.

A gratitude journal is also a great tool. Adding a few entries just before bedtime or first thing in the morning works well. But don't limit your practice to a certain time of day. Start mentally logging entries whenever you think about it—and watch your experience of life improve. Make use of the small moments during each day. With 40,000 thoughts a day, there's plenty of fluff. Certainly you could spare a few dozen for this.

Be patient. Be persistent. A few thankful thoughts in a mind moving at breakneck speed will not bring what you want right away. But as your mind begins to slow down and focus on these thoughts, their power will grow. Just remember that heartfelt gratitude is your immediate goal. If you don't feel it, you're not there yet, but be patient with yourself as these things take root in your heart. It takes a little time. Once you begin to recognize what heartfelt gratitude feels like, it quickly becomes its own reward.

The reason it takes some time between the thinking and the

Gratitude

feeling is that most of us in the Western world don't have a strong head-heart connection. Practicing gratitude is one of the most effective ways to develop one. With practice you'll gain the ability to change your emotional state at will, giving you a high degree of control over your physiology and your life.

Once heartfelt gratitude becomes more commonplace, the expansive state of gratefulness will begin to show up more often. That's the thankfulness/love/timeless/blissful state that Gerald May tried his best to describe at the beginning of the chapter. Some call it the Presence of God. Whatever you choose to call it, you won't find an experience on earth any better. And by the way, at the time Gerald May wrote of his wilderness experience, he knew he was dying of cancer.

Remember that your time here is limited. This will drive you to be thankful for everything. No one and no thing will be with you forever. Appreciate them while you have them. It's the only thing that makes sense.

Find the gift in every situation. If you have trouble finding it, keep looking. If you still have trouble finding it, you may have encountered one of the following roadblocks:

1. Complaining
2. Focusing on the difficulty
3. Feeling you deserve better
4. Complaining
5. Indulging in self-pity
6. Blaming someone else for your predicament
7. Complaining

Complaining only keeps us stuck in whatever we're complaining about. The complaining itself isn't the problem. It's the lack of gratitude our complaints so clearly point to that's the problem.

Chapter Seventeen

Consider everything a gift. Nothing will diminish your experience of life more than thinking you deserve something. Nothing will enhance your experience of life more than considering everything a gift. The following words are from Albert Schweitzer:

> The greatest thing is to give thanks for everything. He who has learned this knows what it means to live. He has penetrated the whole mystery of life; give thanks for everything. Remember to be grateful for life. Consider it a gift.

The Elixir of Life

Gratitude is the elixir of life. Whatever you apply it to grows. It is alchemy of the heart, transforming everything it touches into gold. Can it really bring you everything you want? Let's review:

Gratitude brings you a sense of wealth before you have more money, feelings of happiness before your circumstances change, and effectively increases your blessings by making you aware of the ones you already have. It enhances your health by strengthening the coherence of your cardiac field. It blocks out anger and resentment, further enhancing your health. And it improves your relationships on every level, which enhances your health even more.

You're kinder when you're grateful, you feel better about life, you have more energy, and you'll probably live longer. Considering how tainted the concept of love has become, gratitude may be the easiest most direct route to the heart of God. And if you're dying, which all of us must eventually do, it will make the process easier, less painful, and more peaceful. What more could you possibly want? If a grateful heart is the only price for all this, shouldn't we gladly pay it?

I'm quite convinced that when the end is at hand and we look back on our lives, one of our greatest regrets will be that we weren't thankful enough. Least of all, perhaps, for life itself. No matter when it ends for each of us, or how bumpy the ride, it's quite a privilege. One we take for granted far too much.

There are people with terminal cancer who say that cancer was the best thing that ever happened to them. This is an incomprehensible statement to most. The only way of understanding it is through the eyes of gratitude. A grateful attitude will allow you to find the gift in any circumstance, but what these rare individuals have discovered is that gratitude itself *is* the gift.

Any cancer patient who would say such a thing is living a life of deep gratitude. There is no other explanation. They abide in the life-thanksgiving-love power that May tapped into briefly at the beginning of the chapter. Cancer patients are sometimes driven to it out of necessity, but the rest of us can go there voluntarily if we're willing to make the effort.

Being grateful for your job, family, and a roof over your head, will get you started, but will not take you all the way. When you are grateful for butterflies, running water, rainbows, and toothpaste, you're on the path. When you are grateful for every breath, knowing that the next one is not guaranteed, you have arrived.

In a sense, this is easier for cancer patients because they realize they are living on borrowed time. What the rest of us don't realize is—it's *all* borrowed time. Understanding that on a deep level brings you face to face with the joy that life is meant to be.

When you can abide in this place of deep gratefulness, rather than merely visit occasionally, you have "penetrated the whole mystery of life." There is nothing else to accomplish, nowhere else to go, nothing to do. You own a piece of Heaven, right here on planet earth. And the beauty of it is, you hold it in your heart, where nothing—not even cancer—can take it away.

Chapter Seventeen

An Exercise

At the end of this section you will come to the acknowledgments. Your task is to read them—and then write your own. It is traditional for authors to acknowledge those to whom they are grateful. But we can do that anytime—even without writing a book. We all have a biography. Whether we publish it or not is immaterial. Gratitude is still in order.

We all have those whose help and guidance has been pivotal in making us who we are. Acknowledging them is powerful medicine. Acknowledging it to them directly doubles the dose, so if it is appropriate to share your writing with someone, please do so.

My acknowledgments are a mix of those who have been instrumental in my life, and in the writing of this book. Yours can be anything you want. Mine are in roughly chronological order. Yours can be in no order at all. Begin with whatever comes to you first, and go from there.

Some of those in my acknowledgments are no longer living. I don't necessarily indicate who, because increasingly it makes little difference to me. Those who have passed are still a source of love and support. I feel them with me. Their physical nature is all that's missing.

Remember that gratitude is a meditation, so do the exercise in a quiet place where you're not likely to be interrupted. And don't forget to use everything we've learned. If someone from the past comes to mind, see him or her in your mind's eye as vividly as possible. Remember a time when you were together. How did it feel? Don't just think about them—*be* with them. The more you focus, the more the experience will deepen.

If you acknowledge someone from a current relationship, remember that you won't have them forever. You will have to say

Gratitude

goodbye someday, one way or the other. Keeping this in mind will deepen your appreciation. Be aware of what you're feeling and where in your body you feel it. If tears flow, let them flow. Don't wipe them away. There are no better tears than these.

If book acknowledgments seem dry, it's because we don't feel connected to those the author is thanking. We're sure those people are important to the author, but don't think that has anything to do with us. Few of you will ever meet those in my acknowledgments, but if you look closely, you will recognize them. They're the same people who are in your life—they just wear different faces and go by different names.

When you're finished reading my acknowledgments, put the book down for a few days, pause, and reflect. Write your own when you are ready, then come back and finish up. Don't let it be a one-time exercise. You should do this formally at least once a year. Once a quarter would be better.

Keep them in a notebook and review them periodically. Notice the differences between them as well as the similarities. Your acknowledgments are a living, breathing, being. Each time you commit them to writing is merely a snapshot of a particular moment in time. My list does not include *all* the people I am grateful for. Just the ones that came to me as I was writing the list. There will be recurring players each time you repeat the exercise, but next month your list will look different than it does today.

Revel in this experience, first along with me, and then on your own. There is no better feeling, and no better use of your time than remembering those you love—and who have loved you. ❧

Acknowledgments

To Mom and Dad: You were the foundation of it all. The solid upbringing you provided has been my greatest asset, and I appreciate it more with each passing year. Thanks for so many great memories: the softball, the bowling, the beach, the laughter—and for Lady. How a dog warrants a book acknowledgment forty years after she's gone is something many will not understand. But I know you will.

To Pop, the only grandfather I ever knew: You made me feel special. If there are any other requirements for being a first-class grandfather, I don't know of them.

To Mrs. Hertzler, my high school Latin teacher: You weren't the first adult outside my home to believe in me, but you were the first to make me believe in myself.

To Lana, the love of my life: Who could have guessed all those years ago when I walked into your Latin class how far and wide our journey together would take us? Thanks for being who you are. Thanks for all you do. Thanks for being willing to try again. It's been an amazing run—and the best is yet to come.

To my children, Bryan, Erin, Alex, and Anna: You have been the great joy of my life. I miss the growing-up years, but I love the

Acknowledgments

adults you've become. I'd enjoy hanging out with you even if you weren't my kids. But I'm proud that you are.

To Gary Gay: Where would I be without you? Thanks for your friendship, your wisdom, your infinite patience, and your prayers. You taught me that there is a different way of looking at life, and that what we see with our eyes is not all there is. **And to Sandy:** I always felt your love and support too. Thank you.

To everyone at Naples Radiologists and Naples Diagnostic Imaging Centers (NDIC): I'm grateful for my time with you. It was pivotal for all that was to follow. A special thanks to those in the mammography section at NDIC. Many of us are scattered to the four winds now, but I won't forget our time together. Some of you guessed it would lead to this book, but I never did.

To the staff at Women's Center for Radiology (WCR) in Orlando, FL, my professional home for the last six years: Thank you for your kindness. I love you all. **To Vicki Belmont:** Thanks for your help with everything, related to radiology or not. **To Dr. Susan Curry:** Thanks for so generously sharing your expertise, and for your most valuable feedback on the manuscript.

A special thanks to Michael Brown, I.T. (information technology) at WCR: To say "Thanks for the technical assistance" would be like saying "Thanks for giving me a hand" to the man who just saved you from drowning. Without you, much of this book would still be floating around in cyberspace. **And thanks to you too, Kurt.** Your help was less visible, but no less appreciated.

To Joanne Ellison: Thank you. It may not seem like you did much, but your encouragement and your timely prayer helped get this project off the ground. **Thanks also to Ingrid Ellers:** Your friendship, prayers, and ongoing support helped me get it finished.

To Dr. Dominick D'Anna and staff: Thanks for introducing me to Network Spinal Analysis. And for expanding my horizons. Your

Acknowledgments

contributions to this book have been deeper than you know.

To Akyiaa Azula, intuitive healer: Thank you. What you do is magical—and so are you.

To Cheri Piefke: Thanks for the great picture, the behind the scenes contributions, and your friendship.

To Cathee Poulsen: Thank you for your wisdom, your patience, and your honesty. To say you were my editor is to diminish your contribution. You've been so much more: counselor, friend, sounding board, encourager, writing coach, personal shrink. I don't know if you expected to fill all these roles when you signed on, but I'm glad you did. Thanks for being so good at all of them.

To Mick Silva: Your advice in polishing up the final manuscript was invaluable. Your words made me see things differently. Or was it your prayers?

To Sue Riger: Thanks for the beautiful website, and for such an inspiring book cover. Thanks for doing all the little things necessary to get this project into print. Thanks for being so talented, so positive, *and* so easy to work with. It was a joy.

To everyone who reviewed sections or chapters prior to publication: Thanks so much for your feedback. No writer can see every angle. He or she needs other eyes to help. You were mine.

To Toni Bankston, Moshe Frenkel, David Perlmutter, and Mick Silva, who wrote endorsements: Thank you for taking the time, and for your kind words.

To Jim Gordon: Thanks so much for the beautiful foreword. You put your heart and soul into it and it shows. I am deeply grateful.

To the faculty and staff at the Center for Mind-Body Medicine: Only as the book began to take shape did I realize how much of an impact the Center has had on my life. I love the work we do. Nothing in my professional life has been as gratifying. And I love being connected with all of you. When one laughs we all laugh. And

279

Acknowledgments

when one cries we all cry. There's nothing better than that.

To Lana: On top of *all* your other talents, and *everything* else you do, you took the time to help with the final editing and proof-reading when things got crazy at the end. I've known you for over forty years—and you still amaze me.

Finally, a special thank you to the Borst family in Bann, Germany—especially to Hermann Borst (Opa): As a young Army physician, it was risky taking my wife and two small children with me to what was then West Germany. It was even more risky moving to Bann, a tiny village where few spoke English.

How exceedingly fortunate we ended up next door to you. We didn't understand a word you said that first evening, but your laugh told us all we needed to know. "Who tells jokes to people that don't even speak the same language?" I wondered. It was my first sense that we were about to experience something special.

Thank you for your patience as I struggled to learn the language. I never told you, but my main reason for learning was to be able to talk to you. Thanks for watching over us. Thanks for all the stories. Thanks for "adopting" us into your sizeable family, a place we still belong. And thanks for making me understand how terrible war is—for everyone.

It's hard to fathom all that happened between that first evening and our tearful goodbye four years later. Even after I came home, I never looked at life the same. I've been home nearly twenty-five years now, and you've been gone over twenty—but it seems like only yesterday. I love you, Opa. And I will never forget you. Knowing you changed everything.

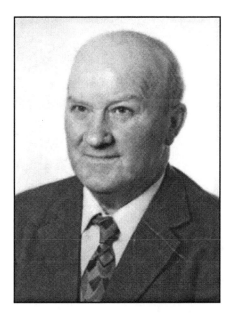

Hermann Borst
1914-1989

Putting It All Together

- No one can take care of you better than you.
- Don't borrow other people's problems. It isn't healthy.
- Know what your doctor can do for you—and what he can't.
- Eat well—and don't stress out about it when you can't.
- Move as much as you can, as often as you can. Your health depends on it.
- Remember that stress is partly self-inflicted.
- Just because you *think* things are a certain way—doesn't mean they actually are.
- Understand what you can change and what you can't.
- Don't waste any time on what you can't.
- No matter what—breathe.
- Focus. There's power in it.
- Be in the present moment. There isn't anywhere else to go.
- Relax.
- Imagine.
- Make sure you imagine something useful.
- If you have a choice between thinking and feeling, always choose feeling.
- Treat your relationships as if they were gold. They are.
- If you need a reason to love someone—it isn't love.
- Learn to listen.

Putting It All Together

- Don't judge anyone. Nothing good ever comes of it.
- A grudge gets heavier the longer you hold it.
- Be patient with yourself.
- Be willing to let go.
- Accept imperfection. It's perfect in its own way.
- Forgive.
- Pray. It doesn't make sense not to.
- Don't *ever* give up hope.
- Don't put God in a box (He won't fit anyway).
- Miracles happen to those who believe in them.
- Focus on health, not disease—especially if you have one.
- Leave your heart undefended. It's worth the risk.
- Cry when you need to; otherwise laugh as much as you can.
- Don't let statistics tell you about you. They aren't smart enough for that.
- Don't lean on your own understanding. There isn't enough of it to hold you up.
- Embrace change. It's going to happen anyway.
- Don't decide anything out of fear.
- If you do, don't be afraid to change your mind.
- Your decisions only have to sit well with you—not with anyone else.
- Don't blame anyone for anything—even if it's their fault.
- Don't complain. It only makes things worse.
- Find your purpose and live it. There isn't time for anything else.
- Trust that there is a higher plan. Know that you will not understand it.
- Enjoy the mystery.
- Don't be afraid to die.
- Be grateful always. This is your reasonable service to God.

෨

Energy Medicine: The Next Frontier

We've touched on the subject of energy in several chapters. It wasn't my intention to do so at the outset of the book, but the deeper implications of the material always led to the same place—our energetic nature. A thorough discussion of energy is beyond the scope of this book, but the subject is important enough to warrant a few words here.

Perhaps the biggest difference between Eastern and Western medicine is that Eastern medicine accepts the reality of the human energy field, while Western medicine does not. Many alternative therapies work by way of the energy pathways in and around the body. Without an understanding of our energetic nature, it is impossible to understand many alternative therapies.

You might think the idea of an energy field surrounding the human body is controversial in Western medicine, but it's not. Controversial, by definition, means somebody's talking about it. But by and large, no one is. As we've seen throughout the book, however, just because there is a prevailing point of view doesn't mean it is correct.

In the modern medical world, the subject of energy faces the same barriers we initially discussed with meditation—preconceived notions and judgments. If an Indian mystic gave a talk about energy to a group of Western physicians, he would get a very different response than Albert Einstein would, even if they gave the same lecture. Resistance to the idea of a human energy field stems from cultural and/or religious paradigms. There is no debate about the science.

The human body works electrically. Electrical impulses and currents are flowing in and around every cell. The heart runs on electricity. The brain and nervous system run on electricity, as do the muscles. In fact, *everything* runs on electricity. "So astounding are the facts in this connection," wrote Nikola Tesla, "it would seem as though the Creator himself had electrically designed this planet."

It is a tenet of basic physics that any electrical current generates an electromagnetic field around it. The earth itself has one, and every living thing on the planet, including humans, has one. Some have called this an aura, a term that is not greeted warmly in scientific circles. But regardless of what you call it, the field does exist. Given what we know about the electrical nature of the body, it *must* exist.

The human energy field, sometimes referred to as the biofield, extends out several feet from the body in every direction. Every piece of information presented to our five senses must first traverse the field, and any type of communication going out must do the same. A good analogy is that of a fish in a fishbowl. Our field is to us like the water in the bowl is to the fish. He is completely surrounded by it. Whatever happens to the water affects the fish, and whatever affects the fish affects the water.

Harold Saxton Burr did much of the pioneering research on biologic energy fields, often referred to as biofields. Burr published nearly a hundred papers on the subject while a professor at Yale University Medical School in the mid-twentieth century. His work culminated in his classic book on the subject, *Blueprint for*

Energy Medicine: The Next Frontier

Immortality: the Electric Patterns of Life, published in 1972.

Burr was convinced that diseases would show up in the energy field before symptoms of pathology would appear. His theory was that if the disturbed energy field could be detected and restored to normal, the pathology could be prevented, an exact parallel of Traditional Chinese Medicine. In 1936 he did a series of experiments on mice that developed mammary tumors, showing that there were large voltage changes detected by electrodes placed on the chest from 10 days to 2 weeks before the tumors appeared.

It is ironic that Western medicine considers energetic healing unscientific, because much of the imaging technology modern medicine relies upon is based on the science of energy. Magnetic Resonance Imaging (MRI) is a good example.

MRI images are produced by placing the person in a strong magnetic field and exposing the body to radio waves. The radio waves "resonate" with hydrogen atoms in the body, causing them all to spin in the same direction. As they relax back to their original, more random, state they emit an energetic frequency of their own, which is picked up by the sensors in the MRI machine and turned into a detailed image. The very fact that MRIs exist is proof that energy waves can cause physical change within the body, *and* that energy waves from the body cause physical change in the "outside world." If it only worked one way, we could never generate an image.

The emerging field of Energy Medicine is based on these same principles. Sometimes physical objects like acupuncture needles are used to move energy. Simply tapping on certain areas of the body with your finger can have a similar effect. Experienced energy practitioners can do the same thing without even touching a person. However the energy is moved, the healing effect can be profound. When decades of stuck emotional energy begins to move, the miraculous sometimes occurs.

Energy Medicine: The Next Frontier

Many hospitals and cancer centers offer energy medicine treatments in one form or another. After having their energies balanced, cancer patients sleep better, have a more positive outlook on life, experience less pain, and have fewer side effects of therapy. Despite their benefit to patients, energy medicine departments are typically understaffed, receive little financial support, and even less support from physicians. If you want these treatments, you'll have to go out of your way to ask for them. But it won't always be that way.

Norman Shealy, M.D., founder of the American Holistic Medical Association, considers energy medicine to be "the future of all medicine." Mehmet Oz, M.D., host of the *Dr. Oz Show*, a daily television show focusing on health issues, has been quoted as saying "Energy medicine is the next frontier." Oz is a major voice helping to bridge the gap between Western and alternative/complementary medicine.

When the medical paradigm shifts, energetic therapies will be there to fill the void. The only thing that hinders this now is the medical mindset. An open-minded look is all that's needed. The science behind it is sound. The following quote is from James Oschman, Ph.D., author of *Energy Medicine: The Scientific Basis*.[1]

> Over the last few decades, scientists have developed more than adequate measurable and logical connections between biological energy fields and generally accepted scientific knowledge. Methods have been developed to measure subtle but important energy fields within and around the human body. A few decades ago these fields were considered nonexistent by academic medicine. Not only are we documenting the presence of such fields, but researchers are understanding how fields are generated and how they are altered by disease mechanisms that enable the discerning therapist to sense and manipulate energy fields for the benefit of the patient.

Energy Medicine: The Next Frontier

An open-minded consideration of energetics has the potential to improve the treatment of serious disorders and diseases that do not respond to clinical methods based on concepts that leave energy out of the picture...Energetic medicine is pointing in an obvious direction...By bringing recent science into the picture, we are finding the missing links in our images of the human body in health and disease.

Whether you have cancer or want to prevent it, you should take advantage of energetic therapies. They have tremendous healing potential and there is virtually no risk. The only downside is that since they are not recognized by the medical system, most aren't covered by health insurance.

You can still take advantage of energy healing, however, even if you don't get formal treatments. Compassion, a grateful attitude, and a positive outlook all have a beneficial effect on the biofield. Our discussion of the cardiac field in chapter 12 makes it clear how much the free flow of our energies depends on us.

Simple forgiveness may be the most effective energy technique on the planet. Many of us carry layers of stuck emotional energy from past hurts. Deep forgiveness releases this, allowing our energies to flow in a more normal pattern. Ah, forgiveness. When it's all said and done—does it really come back to that? ॐ

On a Personal Note

I never set out to write a book—at least not at first. Like many things in life, it "just happened." You make decisions, do what needs to be done, do some things right, a lot of things wrong, struggle with your regrets—and somehow end up right where you were meant to be all along. How does all that work? I have no idea. I only know that it does.

Looking back, I realize that writing was my first love. I spent hours in my room writing stories when I could have been outside playing—and I was an active little boy. When I was eight, I even stuffed some of my stories into a Kleenex box to send off to a publisher. Luckily, when I asked my dad for postage, he convinced me it was a good idea to wait a few decades.

But in the waiting, I forgot. Life happened, which for me included a lot of school, and the writing got lost. Who wants to write when it's required and it's going to be graded? School teaches us much, but important things sometimes get crowded out to make room for all the other important things.

Then suddenly, half a lifetime later, it showed up again—seemingly from out of nowhere. One of those gifts that come out of difficult times. As I began to write down my thoughts and prayers, I found them to be a great comfort. It was like a long-lost friend had unexpectedly shown up at my door.

In many ways this book is a coming out for me. It seems a bit odd at this point in life to finally stand up and say, "Hey, world, this is me; take it or leave it." Ideally we do that a lot earlier in life, but it takes some of us a bit longer, I suppose.

Where do I go from here? I don't know, exactly. Will I write again? Of course I will. When you find your first love again you don't let her go. What will I write? I have no idea—and right now I'm happy not to have one. Like all good things, I won't have to chase it down. It will find me when the time comes.

I've been in your world for a few weeks or so as you've read this book. But you've been in mine much longer than that. As this lengthy project draws to a close, I'm ready for a breather, but I'll miss our daily "conversations." I've wanted to say so much, to so many, for so long; and now I've said it. It's time for what comes next.

No matter what comes next for any of us, it will be helpful to keep in mind what we have learned in *Journey to Hope*. Energy fields, powers of self-healing, and control of our own physiology are not things you will find in mainstream medical books. And yet science proves them to be a present reality. No matter what conventional wisdom might say, they are a firm foundation to build on.

The world works in a fundamentally different way than we ever thought. It is more magical and mysterious than we knew, and we are more wonderful than we imagined. If we think this human existence is one of weakness, we just don't know the rules. With fewer limitations than we knew, we are who we believe ourselves to be, and we can do what we believe we can do. Disease may come, but it is not our master.

What tomorrow will bring, no one can know, but armed with new knowledge, we can face an uncertain future bravely. If we can embrace the mystery, we can live life fully—come what may. To live in such a way, we *must* embrace the mystery, because wonder grows in the same place fear does. Life is not safe. If it were, it would not be worth living.

"It's a dangerous business, going out your door," Bilbo Baggins said to Frodo. "You step onto the road, and if you don't keep your feet, there's no telling where you might be swept off to."

This is where we all step out onto the road. Be blessed on your journey.... ❧

A Prayer

May I spend this day
In humility instead of pride.

May I act out of love
Instead of fear.

May I request,
And not demand.

And be gracious if
My requests are not fulfilled.

May I be gentle.
May I be kind.

May I bring no harm to those
I meet along the way.

May I resist the temptation
To take offense,

And where possible,
Be no offense to others.

May I be quick to encourage
And slow to criticize,

And find a reason to be grateful
In every circumstance.

May I walk in the knowledge
That there is a God who loves me,

And therefore remain in peace,
No matter what this day may bring.

Tom Hudson
July 2011

Notes

Chapter 1: First, a Word to Men

1. Society for Women's Health Research survey: (2005). www.womenshealthresearch.org/site/News2?page=NewsArticle& id=5459 - 51k

2. Kiecolt-Glaser, J.K. (2005). Hostile marital interactions, proinflammatory cytokine production, and wound healing. *Archives of General Psychiatry*, 62(12):1377-84.

Chapter 2: What's My Risk?

1. Feuer, E.J., et al. (1993).The Lifetime Risk of Developing Breast Cancer. *J Natl Cancer Inst*, 85(11):892-7.

2. American Cancer Society. *Cancer Facts and Figures 2009*. Atlanta, Ga: American Cancer Society.

3. Ries, L.A.G., et al. (2004). *SEER Cancer Statistics Review, 1975-2001*. Bethesda, Md: National Cancer Institute.

4. Brinton, L.A., et al. (1988). Menstrual Factors and Risk of Breast Cancer. *Cancer Invest*, 6(3):245-54.

5. Collaborative Group on Hormonal Factors in Breast Cancer. (2002). Breast cancer and breastfeeding: collaborative reanalysis of individual data from 47 epidemiological studies in 30 countries, including 50,302 women with breast cancer and 96,973 women without the disease. *Lancet*, 360(9328):187-95.

6. Henderson, B.F., Pike, M.C., et al. (1984). Epidemiology and risk factors. In: Bonadonna G, ed.: *Breast Cancer: Diagnosis and Management*. Chichester, NY: John Wiley & Sons, pp. 15-33.

Notes

7. Endogenous Hormones and Breast Cancer Collaborative Group. (2002). Endogenous sex hormones and breast cancer in postmenopausal women: reanalysis of nine prospective studies. *J Natl Cancer Inst*, 94(8): 606-16.

8. Colditz, G.A., Rosner, B.A., Speizer, F.E. (1996). Risk factors for breast cancer according to family history of breast cancer. For the Nurses' Health Study Research Group. *J Natl Cancer Inst*, 88(6):365-71.

9. http://www.cancer.gov/cancertopics/factsheet/Risk/BRCA

10. Hollingsworth, Alan B. (2000). *The Truth About Breast Cancer Risk Assessment*, Aurora, Colorado: The National Writer's Press, pp. 45-54.

11. Gail, M.H., Brinton, L.A., et al. (1989). Projecting individualized probabilities of developing breast cancer for white females who are being examined annually. *J Natl Cancer Inst*, 81(24):1879-86.

12. Claus, E.B., Risch, N., Thompson, W.D. (1994). Autosomal dominant inheritance of early-onset breast cancer. Implications for risk prediction. *Cancer*, 73(3):643-51.

13. Smith, R.A. (1999). Risk-based screening for breast cancer: is there a practical strategy? *Semin Breast Dis*, 2.

14. Hollingsworth, Alan B. *The Truth about Breast Cancer Risk Assessment*, p. 5.

15. Eng, S., et al. (2005). Body Size Changes in Relation to Postmenopausal Breast Cancer among Women on Long Island, New York. *Am J Epidemiol*, 162(3):229-237.

16. Bernstein, L., et al. (1994). Physical exercise and reduced risk of breast cancer in young women. *J Natl Cancer Inst*, 86:1403.

17. Matthews, C.E., et al. (2001). Lifetime physical activity and breast cancer risk in the Shanghai Breast Cancer Study. *Br J Can*, 84(7):994-1001.

18. Hamajima, N., Hirose, K., et al. (2002). Alcohol, tobacco and breast cancer--collaborative reanalysis of individual data from 53 epidemiological studies, including 58,515 women with breast cancer and 95,067 women without the disease. *Br J Cancer*, 87(11):1234-45.

19. Helgesson, O., et al. (2003). Self-reported stress levels predict subsequent breast cancer in a cohort of Swedish women. *Eur Journal of Ca Prev*, 12(5):377-81.

20. Lillberg, K., et al. (2003). Stressful life events and risk of breast cancer in 10,808 women: a cohort study. *Am J Epidemiol*, 1;157(5):415-23.

Notes

21. Butow, P.N., et al. (2000). Epidemiological evidence for a relationship between life events, coping style, and personality factors in the development of breast cancer. *J Psychosom Res*, 49(3):169-181.

22. Parkin, D.M., (1989). Cancers of the breast, endometrium and ovary: geographic correlations. *Eur J Cancer Clin Oncol*, 25(12):1917-25.

23. Higginson J., Muir, C.S. (1973). "Epidemiology in Cancer." In: J. F. Holland and E. Frei (eds.), *Cancer Medicine*, Philadelphia, PA: Lea and Febiger, pp. 241-306.

24. Haenszel W., Kurihara, M. (1968). Studies of Japanese Migrants: mortality from cancer and other disease among Japanese in the United States. *J Natl Cancer Inst*, 40:43-68.

25. Dunn, J.E. Jr. (1977). Breast cancer among American Japanese in the San Francisco Bay area. *Natl Cancer Inst Monogr*, 47:157-60.

26. Sorensen T.I., et al. (1988). Genetic and environmental influences on premature death in adult adoptees. *N Engl J Med*, 318:727-32.

27. Lichtenstein P, et al. (2000). Environmental and heritable factors in the causation of cancer: analyses of cohorts of twins from Sweden, Denmark, and Finland. *N Engl J Med*, 343:78-85.

28. http://www.imperial.ac.uk/college.asp?P=3509

29. Lipton, Bruce H. (2005). *The Biology of Belief.* Carlsbad, California: Hay House, Inc., pp. 45-64.

30. Dowley, John E. (2004). *The Great Brain Debate: Nature or Nurture?* Princeton, N.J.: Princeton University Press, pp. 54-56.

31. Lazar, S.W., et al. (2005). Meditation experience is associated with increased cortical thickness. *Neuroreport,* 16(17):1893-97.

32. Waterland, R.A., Jirtle, R.L. (2003). Transposable elements: targets for early nutritional effects on epigenetic gene regulation. *Mol Cell Biol*, 23:5293-5300.

33. Bygren L.O., Kaati G., Edvinsson S. (2001). Longevity determined by ancestors' overnutrition during their slow growth period. *Acta Biotheoret*, **49**:53-59.

34. Kaati G., Bygren L.O., Edvinsson S. (2002). Cardiovascular and diabetes mortality determined by nutrition during parents' and grandparents' slow growth period. *Eur J Hum Genet*, **10**:682–688.

35. Lipton, Bruce H. *The Biology of Belief*, pp. 104-105.

Notes

Chapter 3: The New Medicine

1. Astin, John. (1998). "Why Patients Use Alternative Medicine: Results of a National Study." *JAMA*, 279(19):1548-53.

2. US Dept of Health and Human Services Report on Prescription Drug Importation: (2004).

3. http://www.foxnews.com/story/0,2933,255758,00.html

4. http://www.naturalnews.com/027794_narcotics_addiction.html

5. Lazarou, J., et al. (1998). Incidence of Adverse Drug Reactions in Hospitalized Patients. *JAMA*, 297(15):1200-1209.

6. http://www.photius.com/rankings/healthranks.html

7. http://www.photius.com/rankings/total_health_expenditure_as_pecent_of_gdp_2000_to_2005.html

8. http://nccam.nih.gov/research/camonpubmed/background.htm

9. Richardson, M.A., et al. (2000). Complementary/alternative medicine use in a comprehensive cancer center and the implications for oncology. *Journal of Clinical Oncology*, 18:2505-14.

10. http://www.cancer.org/Cancer/BreastCancer/OverviewGuide/breast-cancer-overview-prevention

11. http://www.webmd.com/search/search_results/default.aspx?query=breast%20cancer%20prevention&sourceType=undefined

12. Bernstein, L., et al. (1994). Physical exercise and reduced risk of breast cancer in young women. *J Natl Cancer Inst*, 86:1403.

13. Matthews, C.E., et al. (2001). Lifetime physical activity and breast cancer risk in the Shanghai Breast Cancer Study. *Br J Can*, 84(7):994-1001.

14. Holmes, M.D., et al. (2005). Physical Activity and Survival After Breast Cancer Diagnosis. *JAMA*; 293:2479 - 2486.

Chapter 4: Self-Care

1. http://www.alternative-cancer-care.com/The_Cancer_Personality.htm

2. Langer, E., Rodin, J. (1976). The Effects of Enhanced Personal Responsibility for the Aged: A Field Experiment in an Institutional Setting. *Journal of Personality and Social Psychology*, 34:191-198.

3. Rodin, J., Langer, E. (1977). Long-term Effects of a Control-Relevant Intervention Among the Institutionalized Aged. *J Per and Soc Psych*, 35:897-902.

Notes

4. Harvey, Lynn K. (1993). Physician Opinion on Health Care Issues (report). (Chicago, Ill.: American Medical Association, May, 1993). p. 21.

Chapter 5: Eat Better, Feel Better, Live Longer

1. Food, Nutrition, and the Prevention of Cancer: A Global Perspective. (1997). *American Inst for Cancer Research.* Washington, DC.

2. Carroll, K.K., et al. (1986). Fat and Cancer. *Cancer,* 58:1818-1825.

3. Verreault, R., et al. (1988). Dietary fat in relation to prognostic indicators in breast cancer. *J Natl Cancer Inst,* 80(1):819-25.

4. Gregorio, D.I., et al. (1985). Dietary fat consumption and survival among women with breast cancer. *J Natl Cancer Inst,* 75(1):37-41.

5. Campbell, T. Colin, and Campbell, Thomas M., II. (2006). *The China Study.* Dallas: BenBella Books, pp. 86-87.

6. Nicholson A. (1996). Diet and the prevention and treatment of breast cancer. *Altern Ther Health Med,* 2(6):32-38.

7. Campbell, T. Colin. *The China Study,* pp. 88-89.

8. Ibid., pp. 65-67.

9. Barley, Lisa. "How Bread is Made," *Vegetarian Times.* March, 2005.

10. Fallon, Sally. (2001). Dirty Secrets of the Food Processing Industry, *Consumer Health,* 24(8).

11. Ibid.

12. Dufty, William. (1975). *Sugar Blues.* New York: Warner Books, p. 216.

13. Sanchez, A., et al. (1973). Role of Sugars in Human Neutrophilic Phagocytosis. *Am J Clin Nutr,* 261:1180-1184.

14. http://www.cspinet.org/new/sugar.html

15. Flegal, K.M., et al. (2002). Prevalence and trends in obesity among U.S. adults, 1999–2000. *JAMA,* 288(14):1723–1727.

16. Haomiao, Jia. (2010). Trends in Quality-Adjusted Life-Years Lost Contributed by Smoking and Obesity. *American J Prev Med,* 38(2):138-144.

17. Eng, S., et al. (2005). Body Size Changes in Relation to Post-menopausal Breast Cancer among Women on Long Island, New York. *Am J Epidemiol,* 162(3):229-237.

18. Enger, S., et al. (2004). Body weight correlated with mortality in early-stage breast cancer. *Arch Surg,* 139(9):954-960.

19. Petrelli, J.M., et al. (2002). Body mass index, height, and post-menopausal breast cancer mortality in a prospective cohort of U.S. women. *Cancer Causes and Control,* 13(4):325–332.

Notes

20. Calle, E.E., et al. (2003). Overweight, obesity, and mortality from cancer in a prospectively studied cohort of U.S. adults. *New England Journal of Medicine*, 348(17):1625–1638.

21. Fuhrman, Joel. (2003). *Eat to Live*. New York: Little, Brown, and Company, p. 119.

22. http://www.hsph.harvard.edu/nutritionsource/what-should-you-eat/vegetables-full-story/

23. Patterson, B.H., et al. (1990). Fruit and vegetables in the American diet: data from the NHANES II survey. *American Journal of Public Health*, 80(12):1443-1449.

24. Fuhrman, Joel. *Eat to Live*, p. 74.

25. Steinmetz, K.A., et al. (1991). Vegetables, fruit and cancer II. Mechanisms. *Cancer Causes and Control*, 2:427.

26. Mettler, Fred A., and Upton, Arthur C. (1985). *The Medical Effects of Ionizing Radiation*. Philadelphia: W.B. Saunders Company, p. 13.

27. Liu, Rui. (2004). Apple phytochemicals and their health benefits. *Nutrition Journal*, 3:5.

28. Eberhardt, M.V., et al. (2000). Antioxidant activity of fresh apples. *Nature*, 405:903-904.

29. Ray, Mitra. (2002). *From Here to Longevity* Seattle: Shining Star Publishing, p. 171.

30. Larsson, S., et al. (2010). Multivitamin use and breast cancer incidence in a prospective cohort of Swedish women. *Am J Clin Nutr*, 91:1268-1272.

31. Smith, M.J., et al. (1999). Supplementation with fruit and vegetable extracts may decrease DNA damage in the peripheral lymphocytes of an elderly population. *Nutrition Research*, 19(10):1507-1518.

32. Inserra, P., et al. (1999). Immune Function in Elderly Smokers and Nonsmokers Improves During Supplementation with Fruit and Vegetable Extracts. *Integrative Medicine*, 2(1):3-10.

33. Food, Inc. (2008). DVD. Robert Kenner (Director). Karl Weber (Editor).

34. http://edis.ifas.ufl.edu/pi180

35. http://www.fromthewilderness.com/free/ww3/100303_eating_oil.html

36. Ibid.

37. Corliss, J. (1993). Pesticide metabolites linked to breast cancer. *J Nat Cancer Inst*, 85:602.

38. http://serc.carleton.edu/microbelife/topics/deadzone/

39. http://www.salem-news.com/articles/april072011/male-breast-cancer-tk.php

40. Personal communication with Jerrol Kimmel, R.N., M.A., Founder of *Filling up on Wholeness: A Whole Person Approach to Well-Being and Weight.* www.jerrol.com

Chapter 6: What About All the Stress?

1. Crow, Michael, executive vice provost for research at Columbia University as quoted in Miracles at Warp Speed. By Bob Herbert, *New York Times* Dec 31, 1999.

2. Wurman, Richard. S. (1989). *Information Anxiety.* New York: Doubleday, p.32.

3. American Institute of Stress. http://www.stress.org/

4. Helgesson, O., et al. (2003). Self-reported stress levels predict subsequent breast cancer in a cohort of Swedish women. *Eur Journal of Ca Prev,* 12(5):377-81.

5. Lillberg, K., et al. (2003). Stressful life events and risk of breast cancer in 10,808 women: a cohort sutdy. *Am J Epidemiol,* 157(5):415-23.

Chapter 7: Take a Deep Breath

1. Lewis, Dennis. (1997). *The Tao of Natural Breathing.* Berkeley, CA: Rodmell Press, p. 42.

2. Rudolph, Rama S., and Hymes, Alan. (2007). *Science of Breath.* Honesdale, PA: The Himalayan Institute Press, pp. 26-35.

3. Kenyon, Tom. (2001). *Brain States.* Lillian Springs, Georgia: New Leaf, pp. 49-53.

4. Lewis, Dennis. (1997). *The Tao of Natural Breathing,* p. 15.

5. Caponigro, Andy. (2005). *The Miracle of the Breath.* Novato, CA: New World Library, pp. 4-14.

6. Weil, Andrew. (1999). *Breathing: The Master Key to Self-Healing.* Audio CD. Sounds True.

Chapter 8: Making Meditation Your Friend

1. Benson, Herbert. (1975). *The Relaxation Response.* New York: HarperCollins, xvi.

2. Ibid., pp.74-5.

Notes

3.   Bujatti, M., Riederer, P. (1976). Serotonin, noradrenaline, and dopamine metabolites in the transcendental meditation technique. *J of Neural Transmission, 39*:257-267.

4.   Bevan, A.J.W. (1980). Endocrine Changes in Transcendental Meditation. *Clin Experimental Pharm and Physiol, 7*(2):75-76.

5.   Carlson, L.E., Garland, S.N. (2005). Impact of mindfulness-based stress reduction (IMBSR) on sleep, mood, stress and fatigue symptoms in cancer outpatients. *Int J Behav Med, 12*(4):278-85.

6.   Carlson L.E., et al. (2003). Mindfulness-based stress reduction in relation to quality of life, mood, symptoms of stress, and immune parameters in breast and prostate cancer outpatients. *Psychosomatic Medicine, 65*(4):571-581.

7.   Astin, J.A. (2004). Mind-Body Therapies for the Management of Pain. *Clin J Pain, 20*(1):27-32.

8.   Spiegel, D. (1989). Effect of psychosocial treatment on survival of patients with metastatic breast cancer. *Lancet, 2*(8668):888-891.

9.   Cole, S., et al. (2001). Time urgency and risk of non-fatal myocardial infarction. *Intl J of Epidem, 30*(2):363-69.

10.   Yan, L., et al. (2003). Psychosocial factors and risk of hypertension. *JAMA, 290*(16):2138-48.

11.   Frantzich Brothers. (2004). *Harmonium.* Audio CD, Track 6. LMR Music. ASCAP, Minneapolis.

12.   Johnston, William, Ed. (1973). *The Cloud of Unknowing.* New York: Doubleday, p. 55-6.

Chapter 9: The Power of Imagination

1.   Spiegel, D. (1989). Effect of psychosocial treatment on survival of patients with metastatic breast cancer. *Lancet, 2*(8668), 888-891.

2.   Rider, M.S., Achterberg, J., et al. (1990). Effect of Immune System Imagery on Secretory IgA *Biofeedback and Self-Regulation, 15*(4):317:333.

3.   Siegel, Bernie S. (1986). *Love, Medicine, and Miracles.* New York: Harper Row, pp. 154-155.

4.   Achterberg, Jeanne. (1985). *Imagery in Healing: Shamanism and Modern Medicine.* Boston: New Science Library/Shambala, p. 56.

5.   Ibid., p. 72.

6.   Simonton, O. Carl, Matthews-Simonton, Stephanie, Creighton, James L. (1978). *Getting Well Again: A Step-by-Step, Self-Help Guide to Overcoming Cancer for Patients and Their Families.* New York: Bantam Books.

Notes

7.   Farah, M.J. (1989). The Neural Basis of Mental Imagery. *Trends in Neurosciences*, 12(10):395-399.

Chapter 10: Understanding Your Emotions

1.   Cooper, Gary L., Ed. (1988). *Stress and Breast Cancer*. New York: John Wiley & Sons, p. 3.

2.   Ibid., p. 4.

3.   Ibid.

4.   Greer, S., and Morris, T. (1975). Psychological attributes of women who develop breast cancer: A controlled study. *Journal of Psychosomatic Research*, 19(2):147-153.

5.   Watson, M., et al. (1999). Influence of psychological response on survival in breast cancer: a population-based cohort study. *Lancet*, 354(9186):1331-1336.

6.   Goleman, Daniel. (1994). *Emotional Intelligence*. New York: Bantam Dell, p. 183.

7.   Rosenberg, Marshall B. (2003). *Nonviolent Communication*. Encinitas, CA: PuddleDancer Press, pp. 43-46.

8.   Pennebaker, J.W., et al. (1988). Disclosure of traumas and immune function: health implications for psychotherapy. *J Consult Clin Psychol*, 56(2):239-245.

9.   Stanton, A.L., et al. (2002). Randomized controlled trial of written emotional expression and benefit finding in breast cancer patients. *J Clin Oncol*, 20(20):4160-8.

10. Krakauer, John. (2009). *Where Men Win Glory: The Odyssey of Pat Tillman*. Random House Audio.

11. Ornish, Dean. (2003). *Love and Survival*. New York: Harper-Perennial, pp. 58-59.

Chapter 11: The Importance of Healthy Relationships

1.   Kiecolt-Glaser, J.K. (2005). Hostile marital interactions, proinflammatory cytokine production, and wound healing. *Archives of General Psychiatry*, 62(12): 1377-84.

2.   Ornish, Dean. (2003). *Love and Survival*. New York: Harper-Perennial, p. 42.

3.   Ibid., pp. 45-6.

4.   Ibid., pp. 40-51.

5.   Ibid.

6.   Ibid., p 61.

Notes

Chapter 12: Spirit and Your Health

1. Caine, Kenneth W., and Kaufman, Brian P. (1999). *Prayer, Faith, and Healing: Cure Your Body, Heal Your Mind, Restore Your Soul.* New York: Rodale, p. 4.

2. McTaggart, Lynne. (2007). *The Intention Experiment.* New York: Free Press, p. 93.

3. Dossey, Larry. (1993). *Healing Words: The Power of Prayer in the Practice of Medicine.* New York: HarperCollins, pp. 295-323.

4. Caine, Kenneth W., Kaufman, Brian P. *Prayer, Faith, and Healing,* p. 4.

5. Ibid.

6. Ibid.

7. Seligman, Martin E.P. (2006). *Learned Optimism: How to Change Your Mind and Your Life.* New York: Vintage Books, p. 15.

8. Ibid., p. 14.

9. Greer, S., et al. (1979). Psychological response to breast cancer: effect on outcome. *Lancet,* 2(8146):785-787.

10. Greer, S., et al. (1990). Psychological response to breast cancer: 15-year outcome. *Lancet,* 335(8680):49-50.

11. Watson, M., et al. (1999). Influence of psychological response on survival in breast cancer: a population-based cohort study. *Lancet,* 354(9186):1331-1336.

12. Visintainer, M., et al. (1982). Tumor Rejection in Rats After Inescapable or Escapable Shock. *Science,* 216:437-9.

13. Beecher, H.K. (1955). The Powerful Placebo. *JAMA,* 159:1602-06.

14. Moseley, J.B., O'Malley, K., et al. (2002) A Controlled Trial of Arthroscopic Surgery for Osteoarthritis of the Knee. *New England Journal of Medicine,* 347(2): 81-88.

15. Kuby, Lolette. (2001). *Faith and the Placebo Effect.* Novato, California: Origin Press, p. 160.

16. Lipton, Bruce H. (2005). *The Biology of Belief.* Carlsbad, California: Hay House, Inc., p.112.

17. Science of the Heart: Exploring the Role of the Heart in Human Performance. (e-booklet) available for free download at: http://www.heartmath.org/research/science-of-the-heart/introduction.html

18. Kornfield, Jack. (2002). *The Art of Forgiveness, Lovingkindness, and Peace.* New York: Bantam Books, pp. 110-1.

Notes

Chapter 13: Risk Revisited

1. Kotsopoulos, J., et al. (2005). Changes in body weight and the risk of breast cancer in BRCA1 and BRCA2 mutation carriers. *Breast Cancer Research*, 7:R833-R843.

2. Campbell, T. Colin, and Campbell, Thomas M., II. (2006). *The China Study*. Dallas: BenBella Books, p. 272.

3. Ibid.

4. Willett, W. (2005). Consumption of fruits and vegetables and risk of breast cancer. *JAMA*, 293(2):183-93.

5. Evans, Joel M. (2005). Nutrition and Cancer lecture: Food as Medicine conference, Center for Mind-Body Medicine. Berkeley, CA.

6. Peto, J., and Mack, T.M. (2000). High constant incidence in twins and other relatives of women with breast cancer. *Nat Genet*, 26:411-414.

7. http://www.imaginis.com/breast-health-news/study-identical-twins-of-breast-cancer-patients-face-high-risk-for-the-disease-dateline-june-25-2002

8. Pedrera-Zamorano, J.D., et al. (2009). Effect of beer drinking on ultrasound bone mass in women. *Nutrition*, 25(10):1057-1063.

9. Holstege, G., et al. (2003). Brain activation during human male ejaculation. *Journal of Neuroscience*, 23(27):9185–9193.

10. http://www.cancercenter.com/complementary-alternative-medicine/laughter-therapy.cfm

Chapter 14: Understanding Mammography

1. US Preventive Services Task Force. Screening for breast cancer: U.S. Preventive Services Task Force recommendation statement. (2009). *Ann Intern Med*, 151:716-26.

2. http://www.acr.org/SecondaryMainMenuCategories/NewsPublications/FeaturedCategories/CurrentHealthCareNews/More/MotivesofMammographyGuidelines.aspx

3. http://www.aacr.org/home/public--media/science-policy--government-affairs/aacr-cancer-policy-monitor/aacr-cancer-policy-monitor---december-/mammography-screening-guidelines-scrutinized-at-congressional-hearing.aspx

4. Evans, K. (2010). Review of the US Preventive Services Task Force's Statement on Screening for Breast Cancer. *JDMS*, 26(1):19-23.

Notes

5. Kopans, D.B. (2010). The Recent US Preventive Services Task Force Guidelines Are Not Supported by the Scientific Evidence and Should Be Rescinded. *J Am Coll Radiol*, 7:260-264.

6. http://email06.secureserver.net/webmail.php?login=1

7. http://www.whitehouse.gov/the-press-office/2010/10/01/presidential-proclamation-national-breast-cancer-awareness-month

8. Kopans, D.B. *J Am Coll Radiol*, 7:260-264.

9. Ibid.

10. Ibid.

11. Tarone, R.E. (1995). The excess of patients with advanced breast cancer in young women screened with mammography in the Canadian National Breast Screening Study. *Cancer*, 75:997-1003.

12. Kopans, D.B. *J Am Coll Radiol*, 7:260-264.

13. American Cancer Society. Cancer statistics 2009 presentation. Available at: http://www.cancer.org/docrootPRO.content. PRO_1_1_Cancer_Statistics_2009_Presentation.asp. Accessed December 6, 2009.

14. Gold, M., et al., (1996). *Cost-Effectiveness in Health and Medicine.* New York: Oxford University Press.

15. Rosenquist, C.J., Lindfors, K.K. (1998). Screening mammography beginning at age 40 years: a reappraisal of cost-effectiveness. *Cancer*, 82:2235-2240.

16. Tengs, T.O., et al. (1995). Five-hundred life-saving interventions and their cost-effectiveness. *Res Anal*, 15:369-390.

17. Cady, B., et al., (2009). Death from breast cancer occurs predominately in among women not participating in mammographic screening. In: ASCO. San Francisco (abstr), 2009.

18. Kopans, D.B. *J Am Coll Radiol*, 7:260-264.

19. Feig, S.A. (1983). Assessment of the Hypothetical Risk from Mammography and Evaluation of the Potential Benefit. *Radiologic Clinics of North America*, 21(1).

20. *Committee to Assess Health Risks from Exposure to Low Levels of Ionizing Radiation, National Research Council of the National Academies, Healthrisks from exposure to low levels of ionizing radiation-BEIR VII, Phase 2.* (2006). Washington, DC: National Academies Press.

21. Feig, S.A. *Radiologic Clinics of North America*, 21(1).

22. Ibid.

23. Ibid.

24. Ibid.

25. Rosenberg, R.D., Yankaskas, B.C., Abraham, L.A., et al. (2006). Performance benchmarks for screening mammography. Radiology, 241:55-66.

Chapter 15: Navigating the Sea of Uncertainty

1. Fawzy, F.L., et al. (1993). Malignant melanoma. Effects of an early structured psychiatric intervention, coping, and affective state on recurrence and survival 6 years later. *Arch Gen Psychiatry,* 50(9):681-689.

2. Gordon, J.S., et al. (2008). Treatment of Posttraumatic Stress Disorder in Postwar Kosovar Adolescents Using Mind-Body Skills Groups: A Randomized Controlled Trial. *Journal of Clinical Psychiatry,* 69(9):1469-76.

3. http://www.cmbm.org/integrative_GLOBAL_OUTREACH/ healing_our_troops.php

4. Goleman, Daniel. (1994). *Emotional Intelligence.* New York: Bantam Dell, p. 181.

5. Dreamer, Oriah Mountain. (2003). *The Call.* Audiobook. SanFrancisco: HarperCollins Publishers.

6. Kelly, Patricia T. (2000). *Assess Your True Risk of Breast Cancer.* New York: Henry Holt and Company, pp. 205-208.

Chapter 16: I Don't Want to Die

1. May, Gerald G. (2006). *The Wisdom of Wilderness.* New York: HarperOne, pp. 30-32.

2. Hanh, Thich Nhat. (2002). *No Death, No Fear.* New York: Riverbend Books, p. 4.

3. Siegel, Bernie S. (1986). *Love, Medicine, and Miracles* New York: Harper Row, pp. 22-32.

Chapter 17: Gratitude

1. May, Gerald G. *The Wisdom of Wilderness.* (2006). New York: HarperOne, pp.43-44.

2. Emmons, Robert A., and Hill, Joanna. (2001). *Words of Gratitude.* Philadelphia: Templeton Foundation Press, p. 17.

3. Emmons, Robert A. (2007). *Thanks!.* Boston: Houghton Mifflin, p. 31.

Notes

4.   Ibid. p. 66.
5.   Ibid. p. 153.
6.   Ibid. p. 117.

Energy Medicine: The Next Frontier

1.   Oschman, James L. (2000). *Energy Medicine: The Scientific Basis.* London: Elsevier, pp. 1-4.

Suggested Reading

Chapter 2: What's My Risk?

Kelly, Patricia T. (2000). *Assess Your True Risk of Breast Cancer.* New York: Henry Holt and Company.

Hollingsworth, Alan B. (2000). *The Truth About Breast Cancer Risk Assessment.* Aurora, Colorado: The National Writer's Press.

Love, Susan M. (2000). *Dr. Susan Love's Breast Book.* Cambridge, MA: Da Capo Press.

Chapter 3: The New Medicine

Gordon, James S., and Curtin, Sharon. (2000). *Comprehensive Cancer Care.* Cambridge, MA: Perseus Publishing.

O'Toole, Carole. (2001). *Healing Outside the Margins: The Survivor's Guide to Integrative Cancer Care.* Lifeline Press: Washington, D.C.

Simon, David. (1999). *Return to Wholeness: Embracing Body, Mind, and Spirit in the Face of Cancer.* New York: John Riley & Sons.

Strand, Ray. (2003). *Death by Prescription.* Thomas Nelson Publishers: Nashville.

Chapter 5: Eat Better, Feel Better, Live Longer

Arnot, Bob. (1998). *The Breast Cancer Prevention Diet.* New York: Little, Brown, and Company.

Suggested Reading

Campbell, T. Colin, and Campbell, Thomas M., II. (2006). *The China Study*. Dallas: BenBella Books.

Dufty, William. (1976). *Sugar Blues*. New York: Warner Books.

Fuhrman, Joel. (2003). *Eat to Live*. New York: Little, Brown, and Company.

Keane, Maureen, Chace, Daniella. (2007). *What To Eat If You Have Cancer*. New York: McGraw Hill.

Pollan, Michael. (2007). *The Omnivore's Dilemma*. New York: Penguin Books.

Pollan, Michael. (2008). *In Defense of Food*. New York: Penguin Books.

Servan-Schreiber, David. (2008). *Anti Cancer: A New Way of Life*. New York: Viking Penguin.

Weil, Andrew. (2000). *Eating Well For Optimum Health*. New York: Alfred A Knopf, Inc.

Chapter 6: What About All the Stress?

Benson, Herbert. (1975). *The Relaxation Response*. New York: HarperCollins.

Cooper, Cary L. (1988). *Stress and Breast Cancer*. New York: John Wiley & Sons.

Eliot, Robert S., and Breo, Dennis L. (1984). *Is It Worth Dying For?* New York: Bantam Books.

Hazard, David. (2002). *Reducing Stress: Natural Remedies for Better Living*. Oregon: Harvest House Publishers.

Kabat-Zinn, John. (2005). *Full Catastrophe Living*. New York: Random House.

Wheeler, Claire Michaels. (2007). *10 Simple Solutions to Stress*. Oakland, CA: New Harbinger Publications.

Chapter 7: Take a Deep Breath

Caponigro, Andy. (2005). *The Miracle of the Breath*. Novato, CA: New World Library.

Lewis, Dennis. (1997). *The Tao of Natural Breathing*. Berkeley, CA: Rodmell Press.

Suggested Reading

Rama, Swami, Ballentine, Rudolph, and Hymes, Alan. (2007). *Science of Breath*. Honesdale, PA: The Himalayan Institute Press.

Weil, Andrew. (1999). *Breathing: The Master Key to Self-Healing*. Audio CD. Sounds True.

Chapter 8: Making Meditation Your Friend

Benson, Herbert. (1975). *The Relaxation Response*. New York: HarperCollins.

Hanh, Thich Nhat. (1976). *The Miracle of Mindfulness*. Boston: Beacon Press.

Johnston, William, Ed. (1973). *The Cloud of Unknowing*. New York: Doubleday.

Kenyon, Tom. (2001). *Brain States*. Lillian Springs, Georgia: New Leaf.

Kornfield, Jack. (2000). *After the Ecstasy, the Laundry: How the Heart Grows Wise on the Spiritual Path*. New York: Bantam Books.

Kornfield, Jack. (2002). *The Art of Forgiveness, Lovingkindess, and Peace*. New York: Bantam Books.

Shapiro, Ed, and Shapiro Deb. (2009). *Be The Change*. New York: Sterling.

Targ, Russell. (2004). *Limitless Mind*. Novato, CA: New World Library.

Tolle, Eckhart. (1999). *Practicing the Power of Now*. Novato, CA: New World Library.

Chapter 9: The Power of Imagination

Achterberg, Jeanne. (1985). *Imagery in Healing: Shamanism and Modern Medicine*. Boston: New Science Library/Shambala.

Chopra, Deepak. (2003). *The Spontaneous Fulfillment of Desire: Harnessing the Infinite Power of Coincidence*. New York: Three Rivers Press.

Maltz, Maxwell. (2001). *The New Psychocybernetics*. New York: Prentiss-Hall.

Murphy, Joseph. (2008). *The Power of Your Subconscious Mind*. New York: Prentice Hall Press.

Suggested Reading

Naparstek, Belleruth. (1995). *Staying Well With Guided Imagery*. New York: Warner Books.

Rossman, Martin L. (2000). *Guided Imagery for Self-Healing*. CA: H.J. Kramer and New World Library.

Rossman, Martin L. (1993). Ch. 17, Imagery: Learning to Use the Mind's Eye. *Mind-Body Medicine*. editors Goleman, G. and Gurin, A. New York: Consumer Reports Books.

Siegel, Bernie S. (1986). *Love, Medicine, and Miracles*. New York: Harper Row.

Chapter 10: Understanding Your Emotions

Childre, Doc, and Rozman, Deborah. (2003). *Transforming Anger*. Oakland, CA: New Harbinger Publications.

Goleman, Daniel. (1994). *Emotional Intelligence*. New York: Bantam Dell.

Gordon, James S. (2009). *Unstuck: Your Guide to the Seven-Step Journey Out of Depression*. New York: Penguin Books.

Pert, Candace P. (1997). *Molecules of Emotion*. New York: Scribner.

Rosenberg, Marshall B. (2003). *Nonviolent Communication*. Encinitas, CA: PuddleDancer Press.

Roth, Geneen. (2010). *Women Food and God: An Unexpected Path to Almost Everything*. New York: Scribner.

Chapter 11: The Importance of Healthy Relationships

Ford, Debbie. (1997). *The Dark Side of the Lightchasers: Reclaiming Your Power, Creativity, Brilliance, and Dreams*. New York: Riverbend Books.

Katie, Byron. (2002). *Loving What Is: Four questions that can change your life*. New York: Three Rivers Press.

Ornish, Dean. (2003). *Love and Survival*. New York: HarperPerennial.

Rosenberg, Marshall B. (2003). *Nonviolent Communication*. Encinitas, CA: PuddleDancer Press.

Valentis, Mary, and Valentis, John. (2003). *Romantic Intelligence*. Oakland, CA: New Harbinger Publications.

Suggested Reading

Chapter 12: Spirit and Your Health

Caine, Kenneth Winston, and Kaufman, Brian Paul. (1999). *Prayer, Faith, and Healing: Cure Your Body, Heal Your Mind, Restore Your Soul.* New York: Rodale.

Childre, Doc, and Martin, Howard. (1999). *The HeartMath Solution.* New York: HarperCollins Publishers.

Dalai Lama. (2003). *The Art of Compassion.* Milan: Sperling & Kupfer.

Dodd, Ray. (2003). *The Power of Belief.* Charlottesville, VA: Hampton Roads Publishing Company.

Dossey, Larry. (1993). *Healing Words: The Power of Prayer in the Practice of Medicine.* New York: HarperCollins.

Dyer, Wayne. (2007). *The Power of Intention.* Carlsbad, CA: Hay House.

Frankel, Viktor E. (1992). *Man's Search for Meaning.* Boston: Beacon Press.

Kuby, Lolette. (2001). *Faith and the Placebo Effect.* Novato, California: Origin Press.

Lipton, Bruce H. (2005). *The Biology of Belief.* Carlsbad, California: Hay House, Inc.

McTaggart, Lynne. (2007). *The Intention Experiment.* New York: Free Press.

Morgan, Marlo. (1994). *Mutant Message Down Under.* New York: HarperCollins.

Pearce, Joseph Chilton. (2004). *The Biology of Transcendance: A Blueprint of the Human Spirit.* Rochester, VT: Park Street Press.

Seligman, Martin E.P. (2006). *Learned Optimism: How to Change Your Mind and Your Life.* New York: Vintage Books.

Tolle, Eckhart. (2005). *A New Earth.* New York: The Penguin Group.

Wattles, Wallace D. (2007). *The Science of Being Well.* New York: Cosimo.

Weil, Andrew. (1995). *Spontaneous Healing.* New York: Fawcett Books.

Chapter 13: Risk Revisited

Campbell, T. Colin, and Campbell, Thomas M., II. (2006). *The China Study.* Dallas: BenBella Books.

Suggested Reading

Cousins, Norman. (1979). *Anatomy of an Illness as Perceived by the Patient.* New York: Bantam.

Chapter 15: Navigating the Sea of Uncertainty

Benson, Herbert, and Proctor, William. (2003). *The Breakout Principle.* New York: Scribner.

Chodron, Pema. (1997). *When Things Fall Apart.* Boston: Shambala.

Chapter 16: I Don't Want to Die

Chopra, Deepak. (2006). *Life After Death: The Burden of Proof.* New York: Harmony Books.

Finley, Guy. (2008). *Fearless Living.* San Francisco: Weiser Books.

Hanh, Thich Nhat. (2002). *No Death, No Fear.* New York: Riverbend Books.

May, Gerald G. (2006). *The Wisdom of Wilderness.* New York: HarperOne.

Siegel, Bernie S. (1986). *Love, Medicine, and Miracles.* New York: Harper Row.

Chapter 17: Gratitude

Daisy, Donna. (2010). *Why Wait? Be Happy Now!* Naples, FL: Barringer Publishing.

Emmons, Robert A. (2007). *Thanks!* Boston: Houghton Mifflin.

Emmons, Robert A., and Hill, Joanna. (2001). *Words of Gratitude.* Philadelphia: Templeton Foundation Press.

Fredrickson, Barbara L. (2009). *Positivity.* New York: Crown Publishing Group.

Losier, Michael J. (2003). *The Law of Attraction.* New York: Wellness Central.

Energy Medicine: The Next Frontier

Burr, Harold Saxton. (1972). *Blueprint for Immortality: The Electric Patterns of Life.* London: Random House.

Suggested Reading

Eden, Donna, with Feinstein, David. (1998). *Energy Medicine.* New York: The Penguin Group.

Gerber, Richard D. (2001). *Vibrational Medicine.* Rochester, VT: Bear & Company.

Hunt, Valerie. (2006). *Infinite Mind: Science of the Vibrations of Consciousness.* Malibu, CA: Malibu Publishing.

McTaggart, Lynne. (2001). *The Field: The Quest for the Secret Force of the Universe.* New York: HarperCollins.

Myss, Caroline. (1996). *Anatomy of the Spirit.* New York: Three Rivers Press.

Oschman, James L. (2000). *Energy Medicine: The Scientific Basis.* London: Elsevier.

Index

Index

Index

Index

Index

Index

Index

Index

Index

Index

Vitamin C, 61, 62, 179, 205
Vitamins, 44, 46, 52, 53, 62
Voice of God, 127

W

Weil, Andrew, 90
Western diet, 53
Western medicine, 74, 91, 123, 124,
    177, 198, 285, 287
    See also Conventional medicine
Wheeler, Claire, 77
WHO, 32, 33, 50
    See also Healthcare rankings
Whole food, 50–64
    concentrates, xx, 61–64
    definition, 50
Williams, David, 111
Woods, Tiger, 167
Working with the breath, 90, 94–95

Y

Yahweh, 93

Z

Zero Point Field, 127

CPSIA information can be obtained at www.ICGtesting.com
Printed in the USA
LVOW120432111011

249925LV00002B/10/P